T0320934

EDITOR'S FOREWORD

This special issue is devoted exclusively to the Community Intervention Trial to Reduce Heavy Smoking (COMMIT). This eight year, $45 million program, sponsored by the National Cancer Institute, is the largest community smoking intervention ever attempted. The eight articles provided here present a comprehensive overview of the project's rationale, intervention, and evaluation plan.

COMMIT is of special interest to health educators because it endeavors to integrate research, community organization, and rigorous evaluation to address a significant world health risk. We are grateful to this issue's co-editors for providing our readers with these articles which emphasize the importance of community mobilization, ownership and partnership in educational intervention as well as the difficulties of balancing standardized research protocols against the need to design interventions suitable to a particular and often unique community setting.

This issue of the Journal is our first devoted to a single topic. Deciding to try this format after more than fory issues may have been influenced by our recent experience at the School of Public Health at the University of Massachusetts in Amherst. As our readers know from our last volume, we are implementing a large-scale smoking intervention study sponsored by the National Cancer Institute to test out the merits of a community-based and community-organized educational intervention versus a mass media-oriented campaign. This ongoing study is taking place in four large U.S. cities: Columbia, South Carolina; Durham, North Carolina; Hartford, Connecticut and Springfield, Massachusetts. Implementing agencies include, in addition to the School of Public Health at Amherst, the Connecticut State Health Department, Benedict College in Columbia and North Carolina Central University. The population in this study differs from COMMIT in being primarily black.

A description of preliminary results of the pilot baseline study related to mass media readership, viewing and listening habits and references on the overall study may be found elsewhere [1, 2].

Int'l. Quarterly of Community Health Education, Vol. 11(3), 169-170, 1990-91

© 1991, Baywood Publishing Co., Inc.

REFERENCES

1. G. Cernada, W. A. Darity, T. L. Chen, A. E. Winder, S. Benn, R. Jackson, and J. Tolbert, Mass Media Usage Among Black Smokers: A First Look, *International Quarterly of Community Health Education, 10*:4, pp. 347-364, 1989-90.
2. E. Stanek, H. Pastides, W. Darity, and M. Elkins, City Directories as Sources of Survey Work in Low and Middle Income Black Communities, *American Journal of Public Health, 80*:8, 1990.

George P. Cernada

ACKNOWLEDGMENTS

The Community Intervention Trial to Reduce Heavy Smoking (COMMIT) is a large scale, multi-site project involving the efforts of many people. The articles in this issue represent the contribution of a host of people beyond the listed authors. Colleagues from the coordinating center, Information Management Services, Inc., National Cancer Institute (NCI), each of the eleven cooperating research institutions, and field staff from each of the eleven intervention sites all deserve to be recognized for their contribution. The COMMIT project contract is supported by NCI.

We are especially indebted to Joseph W. Cullen. Dr. Cullen, as Deputy Director of NCI's Division of Cancer Prevention and Control and Head of the Smoking Tobacco and Cancer Program, was the force behind the initiation of COMMIT and provided support for the trial in its critical formative period. His untimely death is an enormous loss to all those concerned with cancer prevention.

Co-Editors

Edward Lichtenstein, Ph.D.
Oregon Research Institute

Lawrence Wallack, Dr.P.H.
University of California

Terry Pechacek, Ph.D.
National Cancer Institute

Int'l. Quarterly of Community Health Education, Vol. 11(3) 171, 1990-91

© 1991, Baywood Publishing Co., Inc.

INTRODUCTION TO THE COMMUNITY INTERVENTION TRIAL FOR SMOKING CESSATION (COMMIT)

EDWARD LICHTENSTEIN
Oregon Research Institute

LAWRENCE WALLACK
University of California-Berkeley

TERRY F. PECHACEK
National Cancer Institute

For the COMMIT Research Group

ABSTRACT

The Community Intervention Trial for smoking cessation (COMMIT) is sponsored by the National Cancer Institute and involves eleven pairs of communities in North America. COMMIT emphasizes a partnership between the eleven research institutions and their respective intervention communities in developing the structures needed to implement the intervention protocol. We summarize the epidemiological data and describe the prior community interventions that set the stage for COMMIT, and discuss how COMMIT may inform state-wide tobacco reduction demonstration programs. An overview of the articles that describe the COMMIT intervention and evaluation plan is presented.

RATIONALE FOR COMMIT

Goals for Disease Reduction

Thousands of epidemiologic and animal studies have provided conclusive evidence that tobacco use increases a person's risk of developing cancer at a

Int'l. Quarterly of Community Health Education, Vol. 11(3) 173-185, 1990-91

© 1991, Baywood Publishing Co., Inc.

variety of sites; in particular, smoking causes lung cancer [1]. Smoking is also a proven risk factor for cardiovascular disease [2, 3]. The weight of the evidence linking tobacco use to cancer and heart disease is so uniformly persuasive that the Surgeon General of the United States has stated, "Cigarette smoking is the chief, single, avoidable cause of death in our society and the most important public health issue of our time" [1].

Consequently, the National Cancer Institute's "Cancer Control Objectives for the Nation: 1985-2000" [4] identifies a reduction in smoking and use of tobacco products as one of the primary objectives in the goal to reduce cancer mortality by 50 percent by the year 2000. If a reduction in the use of tobacco products can be achieved, thousands of lives can be saved each year. However, the addictive nature of tobacco makes cessation of tobacco use extremely difficult, especially for the heavy user. Significant progress has been achieved in the study of smoking and smoking cessation; nevertheless, major questions exist concerning the most effective methods to reach and involve large number of smokers in the cessation process. The problem is particularly acute for heavier smokers.

The risk of cancer and heart disease among heavy smokers is substantial. Both the 1982 Surgeon General's report, *The Health Consequences of Smoking: Cancer* [1] and the comprehensive review of causes of cancer by Doll and Peto (1981) have reviewed the major prospective studies of the epidemiology of smoking and confirm that middle-aged smokers using twenty-five or more cigarettes per day have a relative risk of lung cancer that is fifteen to twenty-five times greater than for non-smokers. The more recent risk estimates from the American Cancer Society's Cancer Prevention Study II show that these relative risks may have *doubled*, since *all* smokers combined now have an estimated relative risk of over twenty-two for men [3]. These heavy smokers have a similarly elevated relative risk for cancers of the larynx, oral cavity, and esophagus [1]. Additionally, the risks of morbidity and mortality from cardiovascular and respiratory diseases are also dose-related [2, 5] and are highest for the heavy smoker. Heavy smokers represent about one-quarter of all smokers but account for nearly half of all the lung and smoking-related cancers among smokers [1]. Hence, heavy smoking is a pressing public health problem.

Readiness for a Community Approach: Phases of NCI Research

COMMIT is funded by the National Cancer Institute (NCI) and is designed as a Phase IV trial within the NCI's programmatic approach to prevention [6, 7]. Phase I and Phase II research involve developing hypotheses about promising risk reduction strategies and developing needed measures and procedures. Phase III studies are randomized trials in samples of convenience wherein the efficacy of a given risk factor reduction program is evaluated. These are outcome studies comparing different risk factor reduction strategies–e.g., for changes in diet, smoking, or screening behaviors–that are generally familiar to behavioral scientists. Phase IV involves the systematic application of previously tested risk factor reduction programs within randomized trials using large, well-defined population samples drawn from entire workforces, neighborhoods, health care plans or communities. These Phase IV studies normally include an assessment of the impact of the risk factor reduction program on disease rates unless the link between behavioral changes and disease outcomes is very well documented (e.g., as with smoking). Phase V in the NCI approach involves disseminating the risk reduction program broadly enough to have an impact on national disease rates. The American Stop Smoking Intervention Study for Cancer Prevention (ASSIST) described below is an example of a Phase V effort. It is at the fourth and fifth phases that community interventions are most appropriate.

Need for a Community-Based Approach

Community-wide smoking cessation approaches are based upon the assumption that many of the important circumstances supporting smokers' decisions to quit, to initiate quitting, and to maintain abstinence are social circumstances [8, 9]. An important aspect of these community-based intervention strategies is that they provide a sustained intervention effect on a large segment of the smoking population, as opposed to a sporadic high-intensity contact with only a small segment of smokers willing to attend clinic-based programs [10].

A variety of community-wide cessation programs have been conducted (e.g., [8, 11-19]). Often, these smoking cessation campaigns have been mounted as a component of community-wide heart disease prevention studies or other national health promotion initiatives. The early data from these community-based smoking cessation efforts have shown modest success but are generally encouraging. The results from the Stanford 3-Community Study demonstrated an impressive quit rate in the intensive instruction community sample [20] though not for the community which received only the media campaign. However, the feasibility of applying a similar type of intensive intervention protocol in other communities as well as the generalizability of the study design have been questioned [21, 22]. Similarly, results from the landmark North Karelia Study are generally favorable but qualified due to a variety of technical issues [23]. While these early community studies were able to measure some positive smoking cessation effects in cohorts, their inability to demonstrate actual changes in smoking prevalence in the intervention versus the comparison communities make it difficult to draw firm conclusions.

Several recent community-based interventions have shown more definitive population-wide cessation results. The Australian North Coast Program [12] utilized a design similar to the Stanford 3-Community Study, but the evaluation of the community-wide cessation rates was stronger since the effect was measured on independent population samples. The 15 percent net reduction in smoking in that study provides an estimate of the level of treatment effect which can be achieved by a community-based cessation intervention. However, this study suffered from the methodological problem of non-random assignment of communities and a small sample of sites; hence, the results still must be interpreted with caution. Data from the more recent Australian "Quit for Life" media-based campaigns provide a basis for optimism for a sustained anti-smoking effect [17] although the impact was primarily among men [24]. The stronger evaluation methodology of this study increases the confidence in concluding that population-wide effects on smoking prevalence were produced [11].

Preliminary data from the current generation of U.S. Community Heart Disease Prevention trials also are encouraging. Recently published data from the Stanford 5-City Project [25, 26] demonstrate a progressive pattern of smoking cessation in the communities, with the two treatment sites consistently exceeding their matched comparison site during the five-year project. While the quit rate difference between the treatment and control sites within the population-based cohorts increased to 13 percent by the final follow-up, no differences were observed in the independent, cross-sectional surveys of smoking prevalence. The magnitude of changes reported within the Stanford 5-City Project are similar to those projected for COMMIT.

Preliminary data from the Minnesota Heart Health Program [27] suggest that a large proportion of smokers can be recruited to participate in cessation activities and that heavy smokers can be successfully recruited and aided in quitting [8]. While the data analyses of smoking cessation rates in both the Minnesota Heart Health Program and the Pawtucket Heart Health Project [16] are not yet complete, the community heart disease prevention trials have demonstrated that smokers can be reached and involved in community-based cessation programs [8, 28-30].

Smoking's proven status as the major, preventable cause of morbidity and mortality in developed as well as many developing countries around the world makes it the prime candidate for risk reduction interventions. Extensive clinical trial research (Phase III) has yielded a number of promising interventions which can be implemented within specific channels found in a community (e.g., media, worksite, health care providers, schools) while also suggesting that single strategies have limited potential in reaching large populations [31]. COMMIT was initiated in September of 1986 to establish a cooperative intervention trial in twenty-two communities in North America and is the largest smoking intervention trial in the world, involving over two million people. Intervention with heavy smokers (25 or more cigarettes per day) is emphasized due to the greater cancer and cardiovascular risk among this group and difficulty in quitting.

STRUCTURE OF COMMIT

At the national level, COMMIT is a partnership among eleven participating research institutions (one for each site), a coordinating center charged with responsibilities for data management and analysis and logistical support, and NCI program staff. A thirteen-member steering committee composed of the principal investigators from each of the eleven field sites, coordinating center and the NCI project officers, and chaired by an outside expert, is responsible for the scientific management of the trial. The steering committee has an executive committee responsible for overall coordination and charged with handling matters requiring action between steering committee meetings, and three subcommittees to carry out needed work: 1) community organization and intervention; 2) design and evaluation; and 3) publications and presentations. A policy advisory committee composed of national smoking control and health promotion experts is maintained by the NCI to provide broad policy and scientific oversight of the trial and to advise NCI management on trial status and progress.

At the local level, COMMIT is a partnership between the eleven research institutions and their respective intervention communities. The conceptual premise of the trial is that permanent large-scale behavior change is best achieved by community-owned, multi-channel programs that enhance community resources and alter community norms [10, 32-34]. The protocol stipulates that a community board will be formed along with at least four task forces representing the major channels of intervention. Citizen volunteers staff the board and task forces supported by paid staff people hired from the community: a field director, a community organizer, and an office manager. Additional funds are available for materials, subcontracting with local resources, or hiring additional personnel for specific tasks. The number of staff and other resources available to the communities varies according to population and complexity of the local intervention channels.

Figure 1 depicts the organization of COMMIT focusing on the relationship between the research institution and local communities. While no single graphic can accurately portray the actual relationships for all eleven sites, the partnership nature of the organizational structure is a critical element of the trial [35].

PLANNING AND PROTOCOL DEVELOPMENT

During the initial planning and protocol development phase from fall 1986 to summer 1988, trial investigators defined a "state-of-the-art" package of community-based smoking cessation strategies. During the four-year intervention phase which began in fall of 1988, this package is being implemented in all eleven communities. The intervention period will be followed by an eighteen-month phaseout, when data analyses will be performed and final results reported. Figure 2 depicts this overall study timeline.

The intervention protocol was based on prior clinical trials research and focused on four primary intervention channels: public education through the media; health care providers; worksites and other organizations; and cessation resources. Another requirement, consistent with basic tenets of community psychology [36], was that protocol activities be defined such that they largely could be carried out

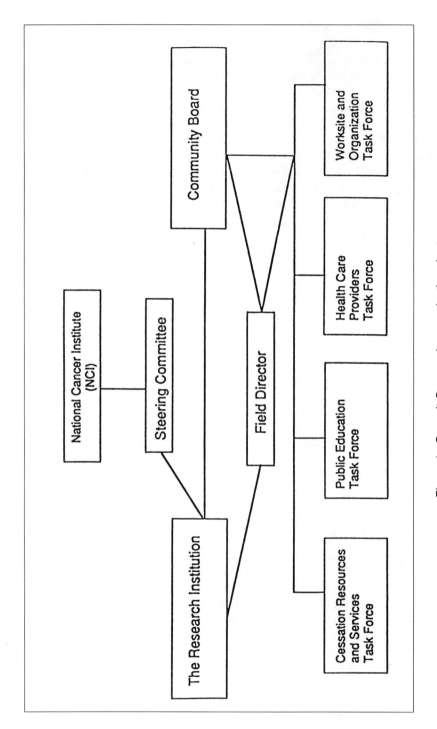

Figure 1. Commit Community organization chart.

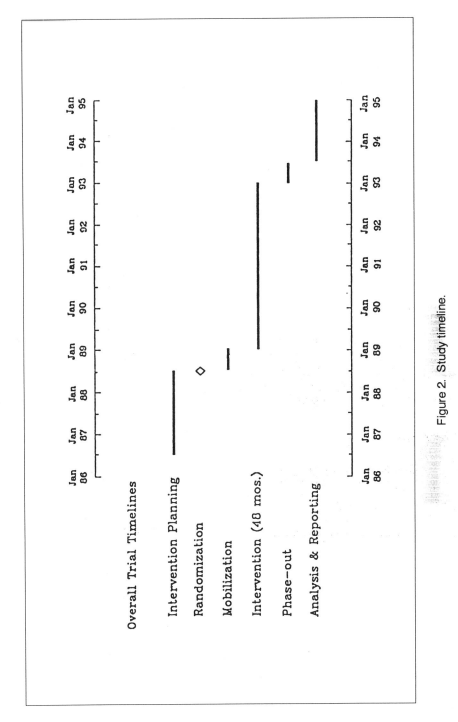

Figure 2. Study timeline.

by community volunteers or local staff or agencies. The research institutions, NCI program staff and other experts provide consultation, training, technical resource materials, and exemplar intervention strategies for the community staff and local volunteers. The decision to emphasize implementation with local resources was guided by the consideration that the *intervention* package being tested must be generalizable to other communities which might not have external resources.

While the research nature of the trial required a standardized level of protocol implementation across all eleven sites, the investigators incorporated a variety of recommendations and protocol adaptations to help communities adopt the protocol to their local conditions [37]. Ultimately, the trial investigators struck a balance between standardization and the principles of community mobilization. Throughout this process, the community and public health aspects of the smoking program were stressed, and are reflected in the trial-wide goals of COMMIT [35]:

- increase the priority of smoking as a public health issue;
- improve the community's capacity to modify smoking behavior;
- increase the influence of existing policy and economic factors that discourage smoking; and
- increase social norms and values supporting non-smoking.

BEYOND COMMIT

COMMIT is a very large scientific undertaking, but it is only one major step toward the ultimate purpose of all of the National Cancer Institute's research on strategies to reduce the use of tobacco: the public health application of proven tobacco control methods [4, 6]. Using the results of its clinical trials and other research efforts, NCI has joined forces with the American Cancer Society to launch the world's largest demonstration project for tobacco control and health promotion ever conducted–the American Stop Smoking Intervention Study for Cancer Prevention (ASSIST).

While COMMIT intervention communities range in size from 57,572 to 163,036, any state, regardless of population, is eligible as an ASSIST site, as are metropolitan areas with a population of at least 2 million. Nevertheless, the organizational structure within an ASSIST site will build upon the COMMIT community mobilization experience [36]. Each ASSIST site is required to form a community-based tobacco control coalition that will be responsible for developing comprehensive tobacco prevention and control plans and implementing these plans in a coordinated fashion throughout the demonstration site. State and local health departments, because of their overall responsibility for the state's or metropolitan area's public's health, will serve as the fiscal agent for the ASSIST coalitions. Within COMMIT, all eleven communities are implementing a common intervention protocol. Within ASSIST, sites will be given more flexibility in the development of their local tobacco prevention and control plans. However, the experience from the COMMIT intervention is being used to develop a set of standards to guide the development of the ASSIST plans. These NCI standards will set minimum levels of emphasis for the ASSIST sites in different program areas, including the health care system; workplaces; schools; civic, social and religious organizations; the media; and the social policy arena.

The full implementation of ASSIST will require a significant investment of staff time and program resources for both the National Cancer Institute and the American Cancer Society. It is anticipated that the project will cost between $100 and $150 million in direct resources over seven years. This does not include the vast amounts of volunteer and other in-kind support that will be required in order to make ASSIST truly effective. COMMIT represents the last major tobacco control research effort to be conducted by NCI before ASSIST goes into full implementation. Therefore, COMMIT and ASSIST investigators will need to work closely together through the 1990s to insure that the results from COMMIT are fully prepared for national dissemination.

OVERVIEW OF SPECIAL ISSUE PAPERS

A central feature of COMMIT is the active involvement of citizens and community organizations in planning and delivering intervention activities. In the first article, Beti Thompson and colleagues describe the development and implementation of the protocol that guides community mobilization [35]. Standardizing this portion of the protocol, given the diversity of communities, was a considerable challenge. Stipulating a common endpoint organizational structure–a Community Board and four task forces–proved to be a useful strategy in meeting this challenge. Each task force represents a major intervention channel and these are described in the following four articles.

Public education with a major focus on use of mass media is one of the major intervention channels for COMMIT. Lawrence Wallack and Russ Sciandra describe this portion of the protocol and present several examples of how communities have creatively exploited national and local events in the service of COMMIT goals [38]. Wallack and Sciandra also describe the emerging strategy of media advocacy and discuss some of the issues surrounding the use of this more confrontational approach to media use in COMMIT sites.

Baseline survey data from the COMMIT sites showed that over 70 percent of smokers see a health care provider once a year or more and perceive them as credible sources of health information. Therefore, health care providers and settings are a major channel for COMMIT interventions. Judith Ockene and colleagues describe the extensive health care setting portion of the protocol and present several examples of how communities have implemented activities [39].

Worksites and other community organizations represent the third major COMMIT intervention channel since 70 percent of the adults in the COMMIT sites are in the workforce. Glorian Sorensen and colleagues describe the worksite portion of the protocol describing the major worksite policy, motivational, and cessation facilitating activities defined in the trial protocol [40]. They present data from baseline evaluation surveys depicting variability across communities in current policies. Further data on size of worksites points out another challenge for COMMIT: addressing the numerous small worksites that contain the majority of smokers.

Cessation services are an important part of any community approach to smoking reduction. Paul Pomrehn and colleagues describe the cessation resources portion of the protocol [41]. The two major components–smokers network and local, tailored cessation resources guides–are integrated with the other three major channels (media, health care provider, worksites) in order to provide assistance to motivated smokers.

Two articles focus on design and evaluation issues. Over one-half of the COMMIT budget goes to research and evaluation. Margaret Mattson and colleagues summarize the research design and major evaluation strategies and procedures [42]. As this article shows, COMMIT is the first community trial using a matched pairs design, with communities as both the unit of assignment and analysis, that has *adequate* statistical power to detect differences in quit rates. Procedures for assessing outcome, impact, and process objectives also are described. Additionally, examples are presented of how some of the data are being used to inform the intervention.

In a complementary article on process evaluation, Kitty Corbett and colleagues describe in detail the procedures for monitoring community mobilization and intervention activities [43]. Determining how well communities are implementing the protocol is critical for management and evaluation purposes. The procedures described by Corbett et al. will permit an analysis of how and why intervention did or did not work.

In their collectivity, the articles in this issue provide both a broad and intensive account of the largest smoking cessation trial ever undertaken. The methodologies employed and the emphasis on community participation are likely to serve as models for a variety of other future health promotion efforts.

REFERENCES

1. U.S. Department of Health and Human Services, *The Health Consequences of Smoking: Cancer. A Report of the Surgeon General* (DHHS Publication No. PHS 82-50179), Public Health Service, Office on Smoking and Health, Washington, D.C., 1982.
2. U.S. Department of Health and Human Services, *The Health Consequences of Smoking: Cardiovascular Disease. A Report of the Surgeon General* (DHHS Publication No. PHS 84-50204), Public Health Service, Office on Smoking and Health, Washington, D.C., 1983.

3. U.S. Department of Health and Human Services, *Reducing the Health Consequences of Smoking: 25 Years of Progress* (DHHS Publication No. CDC 89-8411), Public Health Service, Office on Smoking and Health, Washington, D.C, 1989.

4. P. Greenwald and E. J. Sondik, Cancer Control Objectives for the Nation: 1985-2000, *National Cancer Institute Monographs, 2*, pp. 1-93, Washington, D.C., 1986.

5. U.S. Department of Health and Human Services, *The Health Consequences of Smoking: Chronic Obstructive Lung Disease. A Report of the Surgeon General* (DHHS Publication No. PHS 84-50205), Public Health Service, Office on Smoking and Health, Washington, D.C., 1984.

6. J. W. Cullen, A Rationale for Health Promotion in Cancer Control, *Preventive Medicine, 15*, pp. 442-450, 1986.

7. P. Greenwald and J. W. Cullen, The New Emphasis in Cancer Control, *Journal of the National Cancer Institute, 74*, pp. 543-551, 1985.

8. H. Blackburn and T. F. Pechacek, Smoking Cessation and the Minnesota Heart Health Program, in *Proceedings of the Fifth World Conference on Smoking and Health, 2*, pp. 159-164, W. F. Forbes, R. C. Frecker, and D. Nostbakken (eds.), Canadian Council on Smoking and Health, Ottawa, Canada, 1986.

9. J. W. Farquhar, P. F. Magnus, and N. Maccoby, The Role of Public Information and Education in Cigarette Smoking Controls, *Canadian Journal of Public Health, 72*:2, pp. 412-420, 1981.

10. L. Green and A. McAlister, Macro-Intervention to Support Health Behavior: Some Theoretical Perspectives and Practical Reflections, *Health Education Quarterly, 11*, pp. 322-339, 1984.

11. T. Dwyer, J. P. Pierce, and C. D. Hannan, Evaluation of the Sydney "Quit for Life" Anti-Smoking Campaign. Part 2, Changes in Smoking Prevalence, *Medical Journal of Australia, 144*, pp. 344-347, 1986.

12. G. Effer, W. Fitzgerald, G. Frape, A. Monaem, P. Rubinstein, C. Tyler, and B. McKay, Results of Large-Scale Media Anti-Smoking Campaign in Australia: North Coast "Quit for Life" Programme, *British Medical Journal, 287*, pp. 1125-1128, 1983.

13. J. W. Farquhar, S. P. Fortmann, N. Maccoby, et al., The Stanford Five City Project: An Overview, in *Behavioral Health: A Handbook of Health Enhancement and Disease Prevention*, J. D. Matarazzo, S. M. Weiss, J. A. Herd, N. E. Miller, and S. M. Weiss (eds.), John Wiley & Sons, New York, pp. 1154-1165, 1984.

14. B. R. Flay, Mass Media and Smoking Cessation: A Critical Review, *American Journal of Public Health, 77*:2, pp. 153-160, 1987.

15. M. Kornitzer, M. Dramaix, F. Kittel, and G. DeBacker, The Belgian Heart Disease Prevention Project: Changes in Smoking Habits after Two Years of Intervention, *Preventive Medicine, 9*:4, pp. 496-503, 1980.

16. T. Lasater, D. Abrams, L. Artz, et al., Lay Volunteer Delivery of a Community-Based Cardiovascular Risk Factor Change Program: The Pawtucket Experiment, in *Behavioral Health: A Handbook of Health Enhancement and Disease Prevention*, J. D. Matarazzo, S. M. Weiss, J. A. Herd, N. E. Miller, and S. M. Weiss (eds.), John Wiley & Sons, New York, pp. 1166-1170, 1984.

17. J. P. Pierce, T. Dwyer, G. Frape, S. Chapman, A. Chamberlain, and N. Burke, Evaluation of the Sydney "Quit for Life" Antismoking Campaign. Part 1. Achievement of Intermediate Goals, *Medical Journal of Australia, 144*, pp. 341-347, 1986.

18. P. Puska and K. Koskela, Community-Based Strategies to Fight Smoking: Experiences from the North Karelia Project in Finland, *New York State Journal of Medicine, 84*, pp. 1135-1138, 1983.
19. R. E. Rice and C. K. Atkin (eds.), *Public Communication Campaigns*, (2nd Edition), Sage Publications, Newbury Park, California, 1989.
20. J. W. Farquhar, P. D. Wood, H. Breitrose, et al., Community Education for Cardiovascular Health, *Lancet, 1*:8023, pp. 1192-1195, 1977.
21. S. V. Kasl, Cardiovascular Risk Reduction in a Community Setting: Some Comments, *Journal of Consulting and Clinical Psychology, 48*:2, pp. 143-149, 1980.
22. H. Leventhal, P. D. Cleary, M. A. Safer, and M. Gutmann, Cardiovascular Risk Modification by Community-Based Programs for Life-Style Change: Comments on the Stanford Study, *Journal of Consulting and Clinical Psychology, 48*:2, pp. 150-158, 1980.
23. P. Puska, Community-Based Prevention of Cardiovascular Disease: The North Karelia Project, in *Behavioral Health: A Handbook of Health Enhancement and Disease Prevention*, Wiley & Sons, Inc., New York, pp. 1140-1147, 1984.
24. J. P. Pierce, P. Macaskill, and D. Hill, Long-Term Effectiveness of Mass Media Led Antismoking Campaigns in Australia, *American Journal of Public Health, 80*:5, pp. 565-569, 1990.
25. J. W. Farquhar, S. P. Fortmann, N. Maccoby, et al., The Stanford Five-City Project: Design and Methods, *American Journal of Epidemiology, 122*, pp. 323-334, 1985.
26. J. W. Farquhar, S. P. Fortmann, J. A. Flora, D. B. Taylor, et al., Effects of Community-Wide Education on Cardiovascular Disease Risk Factors, *Journal of the American Medical Association, 264*:3, pp. 359-365, 1990.
27. H. Blackburn, R. V. Luepker, F. G. Kline, et al., The Minnesota Heart Health Program: A Research and Demonstration Project in Cardiovascular Disease Prevention, in *Behavioral Health: A Handbook of Health Enhancement and Disease Prevention*, J. D. Matarazzo, S. M. Weiss, J. A. Herd, N. E. Miller, and S. M. Weiss (eds.), John Wiley & Sons, New York, pp. 1171-1178, 1984.
28. D. Altman, J. Flora, S. P. Fortmann, and J. W. Farquhar, The Cost-Effectiveness of Three Smoking Cessation Programs, *American Journal of Public Health, 77*, pp. 162-165, 1987.
29. J. P. Elder, S. A. McGraw, A. Rodriques, T. M. Lasater, et al., Evaluation of Two Community-Wide Smoking Cessation Contests, *Preventive Medicine, 16*, pp. 221-234, 1987.
30. J. R. Finnegan, D. M. Murray, C. Kurth, and P. McCarthy, Measuring and Tracking Education Program Implementation: The Minnesota Heart Health Program Experience, *Health Education Quarterly, 16*:1, pp. 77-90, 1989.
31. National Cancer Institute, *The Smoking, Tobacco, and Cancer Program: 1985-1989 Status Report* (DHHS Publication No. NIH 90-3107), U.S. Government Printing Office, Washington, D.C., 1990.
32. N. Bracht (ed.), *Health Promotion at the Community Level*, Sage Publications, Newbury Park, California, 1990.
33. R. Carlaw, M. Mittelmark, N. Bracht, and R. Luepker, Organization for a Community Cardiovascular Health Program: Experiences from the Minnesota Heart Health Program, *Health Education Quarterly, 11*, pp. 243-252, 1984.

34. A. McAlister, P. Puska, J. Salonen, J. Tuomilehto, and K. Koskela, Theory and Action for Health Promotion: Illustrations from the North Karelia Project, *American Journal of Public Health, 72*, pp. 43-50, 1982.
35. B. Thompson, L. Wallack, E. Lichtenstein, and T. Pechacek, Principles of Community Organization and Partnership for Smoking Cessation in the Community Intervention Trial to Reduce Heavy Smoking (COMMIT), *International Quarterly of Community Health Education, 11*:3, pp. 187-203, 1990-91.
36. E. Lichtenstein, L. Nettekoven, and J. K. Ockene, Community Intervention Trial for Smoking Cessation (COMMIT): Opportunities for Community Psychologists in Chronic Disease Prevention, Manuscript submitted for publication, 1990.
37. B. Thompson and R. Karmi, *A Handbook for Community Change*, National Cancer Institute, Washington, D.C., 1988.
38. L. Wallack and R. Sciandra, Media Advocacy and Public Education in the Community Intervention Trial to Reduce Heavy Smoking (COMMIT), *International Quarterly of Community Health Education, 11*:3, pp. 205-222, 1990-91.
39. J. K. Ockene, E. L. Lindsay, L. Berger, and N. Hymowitz, Health Care Providers as Key Change Agents in the Community Intervention Trial for Smoking Cessation (COMMIT), *International Quarterly of Community Health Education, 11*:3, pp. 223-237, 1990-91.
40. G. Sorensen, R. E. Glasgow, and K. Corbett, Promoting Smoking Control through Worksites in the Community Intervention Trial for Smoking Cessation (COMMIT), *International Quarterly of Community Health Education, 11*:3, pp. 239-257, 1990-91.
41. P. Pomrehn, R. Sciandra, R. Shipley, W. Lynn, and H. Lando, Enhancing Resources for Smoking Cessation through Community Intervention: COMMIT as a Prototype, *International Quarterly of Community Health Education, 11*:3, pp. 259-269, 1990-91.
42. M. E. Mattson, K. M. Cummings, W. R. Lynn, C. Giffen, D. Corle, and T. Pechacek, Evaluation Plan for the Community Intervention Trial for Smoking Cessation (COMMIT), *International Quarterly of Community Health Education, 11*:3, pp. 271-290, 1990-91.
43. K. Corbett, B. Thompson, N. White, and M. Taylor, Process Evaluation in the Community Intervention Trial for Smoking Cessation (COMMIT), *International Quarterly of Community Health Education, 11*:3, pp. 291-309, 1990-91.

Direct reprint requests to:

Edward Lichtenstein, Ph.D.
Oregon Research Institute
1899 Willamette Street
Eugene, OR 97401

PRINCIPLES OF COMMUNITY ORGANIZATION AND PARTNERSHIP FOR SMOKING CESSATION IN THE COMMUNITY INTERVENTION TRIAL FOR SMOKING CESSATION (COMMIT)

BETI THOMPSON
Fred Hutchinson Cancer Research Center
University of Washington, Seattle

LAWRENCE WALLACK
University of California, Berkeley

EDWARD LICHTENSTEIN
Oregon Research Institute, Eugene

TERRY PECHACEK
National Cancer Institute, Bethesda, Maryland

For the COMMIT Research Group

ABSTRACT

The Community Intervention Trial for Smoking Cessation (COMMIT) has adopted a community approach to smoking cessation. State-of-the-art interventions that have proven efficacious for smoking cessation are delivered to smokers through community-based organizations. An innovative adaptation of community organization methods accommodated the need for a standardized protocol with the flexibility required for diverse and unique communities. The unique characteristics of the eleven intervention communities are examined with a focus on differences in size, location, availability and importance of the intervention channels, and other factors that were important for community mobilization. Initial results of the mobilization process are summarized. Although there were some differences in the structures formed and the time required to complete the initial project activities, all eleven intervention sites were mobilized around the COMMIT goals and activities.

Int'l. Quarterly of Community Health Education, Vol. 11(3) 187-203, 1990-91

© 1991, Baywood Publishing Co., Inc.

Smoking continues to be a major cause of premature death and disability in our society [1, 2]. The United States' National Cancer Institute, in an ambitious effort to achieve a widespread reduction in the prevalence of smoking, launched an extensive research project, the Community Intervention Trial for Smoking Cessation (COMMIT), to assess the effectiveness of a comprehensive community-based effort to help all smokers, and especially heavy smokers, to achieve and maintain smoking cessation.

One unique attribute of COMMIT is its reliance on a community-based approach to smoking cessation. Traditional approaches to smoking cessation have focused on the individual, with little attention given to the broader social context within which that individual acts. A great deal has been accomplished at that individual level and certainly, many people have been convinced to make behavior changes around smoking [3, 4]. Increasingly, however, there is a recognition that the decision to smoke takes place in a complex web of formal and informal policies and actions that reflect community norms and values [5-8]. An important feature of the COMMIT trial is the move to a community level intervention designed to influence not only individuals, but also the broader social context.

Four major aspects of the community approach utilized by COMMIT are reviewed in this article. They include the rationale for a community approach, the principles of community partnership adopted by COMMIT, the balance struck between local versus trial-wide influence, and a review of the early community mobilization experiences of the eleven sites.

THE RATIONALE FOR A COMMUNITY APPROACH

There are several reasons that COMMIT is using a community approach to achieve smoking cessation. To achieve a large reduction in smoking prevalence, it is necessary to expose many smokers to both messages about and opportunities for cessation [9]. Clinical programs are limited in the numbers of people that can be reached [3, 4]. Cessation efforts conducted in organizations such as worksites, while reaching more smokers, frequently have relatively low participation rates [10]. A community approach has greater potential for reaching large numbers of people [3, 9, 11]. Organizing an entire community around a health promotion project or effort will necessarily involve more people than individual or small group recruitment activities. The reach is further enhanced when messages about behavior change are widespread throughout the community, and it becomes difficult to avoid exposure to them.

Community approaches are likely to involve diverse individuals, groups, organizations, and institutions [9, 12, 13]. This kind of involvement provides a greater base for support of the behavior change. Over time, the unhealthy behavior is no longer seen as merely an individual problem; rather, the community takes on some of the responsibility. Examples of this can be found in alcohol control projects, where communities have organized themselves to use policy approaches to change the social and physical environment through which alcohol is made available [14, 15]. This extends the focus to include key factors external to the person as well as individual variables.

The greater base of community support may reduce the funding level required for intervention activities. Community members and organizations can be expected to volunteer time, provide contributed services as well as funds, and distribute responsibility for various intervention activities. The relatively small amount of "seed money" provided by governmental funding agencies is greatly magnified within the community setting, and smoking control activities can be added or integrated into the agendas and programs of agencies with little or no additional resources.

Most importantly, the interventions can be integrated into the community and its institutions so that long-term change is likely [5, 16, 17]. Interventions conducted through community groups and organizations can, with careful planning, become part of the community's resources and services and, thus, endure beyond a governmentally funded intervention period.

For COMMIT, the major impetus for, and underlying assumption behind, the community approach to behavior change is the recognition that behavior is greatly influenced by the environment in which it occurs [8]. Smoking is both cued and constrained by environmental factors. Changing the behavior without changing the cues and constraints may result in difficulty in maintaining the change–putting individuals back into the situation may result in them reverting back to the undesired behavior. Many of the cues and constraints around smoking behavior can be traced to societal norms; that is, shared rules and expectations for behavior [18]. The community approach to health promotion is based on the notion that long-term behavior change is best achieved by changing norms about the behavior.

The trial-wide goals of COMMIT were designed with the view of changing the community environment. Specifically, the goals are to:

1. *Increase the priority of smoking as a public health issue.* Smoking tends to be seen as an individual smoker's issue. This narrow definition of the problem results in clinically oriented cessation programs rather than efforts that stimulate widespread citizen participation and involvement of the major social institutions within a community. A critical step in the COMMIT project is to redefine the smoking problem as a community issue, requiring community as well as individual approaches. An example is found in the way that smoking detracts from the quality of life in the community (e.g., risk to nonsmokers from second-hand smoke; increased morbidity and mortality; loss of productivity); all community members can gain from strategies designed to reduce smoking levels. Because the community shares in the benefits, all community members have reason to participate in the process.

2. *Increase the community capacity to modify smoking behavior.* Because of the emphasis on the individual, community activities to enable smokers to achieve cessation tend to be fragmented and relatively sparse. To encourage and support those who want to stop smoking, the community must have an adequate system of smoking cessation resources and services available. The resources and services must be diverse enough to offer all smokers the cessation method of their choice (e.g., clinical programs, counseling, hypnosis, self-help materials); furthermore, a system of disseminating information about cessation methods must be widely available so that community members can refer smokers to appropriate services. It is not sufficient, however, to increase clinical programs; rather, communities are encouraged to build smoking cessation opportunities and assistance into regular activities that occur within the various sectors of a community (e.g., worksites, organizations, schools). In addition, increasing the community capacity to modify smoking behavior requires an emphasis on prevention as well as cessation; thus, an important piece of the COMMIT project is to incorporate smoking prevention education into a wide variety of youth activities.

3. *Increase the influence of existing policy and economic factors within a community that discourages smoking.* Increasingly, communities and various sectors of communities are implementing policies that restrict smoking [19]. Such policies are very influential in changing the social environment and may have an impact on smokers' decisions to attempt cessation. COMMIT recognizes the contribution policy changes can make for the entire community and advocates such changes. Economic and policy factors within a community that may influence smoking rates include taxation, advertising and promotional restrictions, and restrictions on the sale of cigarettes, especially to minors [20, 21].

4. *Increase social norms and values supporting nonsmoking.* As the trend toward smoking control increases nationally, a norm supporting nonsmoking is emerging; however, progress is somewhat hampered by the still prevalent emphasis on smoking as an individual issue. As it becomes clearer that all community members–smokers and nonsmokers alike–are affected by smoking, opportunities will arise to foster the perception that nonsmoking is normative and to be valued. An essential feature of COMMIT is to build into all activities the explicit recognition that nonsmoking is appropriate and smoking is not.

PRINCIPLES OF COMMUNITY PARTNERSHIP

COMMIT builds on a community organization perspective [22-27]. The basic premises of this perspective make it especially appealing for achieving the widespread change sought in COMMIT. First, basic postulates of this perspective are that behavior occurs within a social context, that large-scale change requires that the social context be changed, and that change is more likely to occur when the people affected by a problem are involved in defining and solving the problem [23, 25, 26]. This latter premise is reflected in the principle of "ownership," important both theoretically and in practice [28, 29]. Essentially, it means that outside "experts"–health educators, researchers, and other professionals–are meant to be facilitators to guide change, not to control and define it. COMMIT, because of its research emphasis, has found it necessary to modify some aspects of the principle of ownership, and the relationships between the communities and the research institutions guiding the project might better be termed a "partnership" [12, 13].

The principle of partnership is reflected in a number of key guidelines for establishing working relations with communities. These tenets are critical for effective and long-lasting community involvement. The first "rule" is that it is important to have real collaboration, not merely representation. An equal partnership means that community members are involved in the whole project and have significant decision-making capability. COMMIT activities that achieve this goal are concentrated in community decisions around implementation of activities and internal allocation of a community budget for conducting the activities.

It is also critical to build on existing community structures rather than replacing or adding new structures that are unlikely to be sustained after external funding expires. It is equally important to work with a community, not in competition with it nor with agencies within it; thus, it is unwise to create something that can be perceived as a threat to existing groups. COMMIT seeks to enhance relationships with ongoing community groups to build the groups' capacity to address smoking control. Such capacity building may include the provision of resources to expand smoking control activities to a wider spectrum of community groups, train cessation service providers, or produce media campaigns to familiarize citizens with smoking control opportunities and activities.

To address a community problem requires long-term planning as opposed to short-term problem solving. For a long-term effect, attention must be paid to underlying factors that influence behavior. For example, the task of educating those at risk to become nonsmokers is substantially easier when the community is structured to promote smoke-free environments. Smoke-free workplaces and public areas, widespread availability of cessation opportunities, and enforcement of rules restricting access to tobacco products by minors all contribute to reinforcing the basic smoke-free message and strengthening educational efforts. Thus, COMMIT seeks to enhance existing community resources available to deal with smoking control, rather than restricting its activities to a single massive recruitment of current smokers into cessation programs.

Another guideline requires that care be taken to recognize community inhibiting and facilitating factors to ensure that the solutions developed are suitable for a community. Communities differ in values, norms, and structures, and those differences are vital to the manner in which partnerships must be established, as well as specific intervention activities. Similarly, there may be unique opportunities in

Table 1. Selected Facilitators and Inhibitors for Community Change
in the Eleven Intervention Communities

Characteristic	Number of Sites Reporting
Facilitators	
Cooperative environment for community improvement	8
Supportive health care environment	7
History of volunteerism	6
Active citizen participation in community leadership	6
Supportive media	5
Experience with coalitions	4
Strong voluntary organizations	4
Existing tobacco-control programs	3
Inhibitors	
Community tension	7
Economic worries	6
Media problems	5
Lack of strong voluntary groups	5
Strong individualism	5
Competing issues	4
Worksite concerns	4
Conservatism around change	3
Pro-tobacco groups	3

a community that will make community organization and interventions easier. A comprehensive community analysis was undertaken by COMMIT sites so that those factors could be identified. As can be seen in Table 1, communities differed extensively in factors identified as potentially inhibiting or facilitating project activities.

More than half of the communities had a strong history of volunteerism on which they can base their COMMIT activities. Four communities had much past experience with coalitions: a history that was likely to enable them to more easily form coalitions for the purpose of smoking control activities. Other facilitators stressed a cooperative or supportive environment for various community sectors. Inhibitors included nonsmoking-related factors such as ongoing community tension, competing issues, and concerns about specific sectors. In addition, three communities had strong pro-tobacco groups.

The approach should be multi-dimensional; that is, it must involve all major community sectors in a variety of ways. It is insufficient to change a single sector of the community and expect the entire community to change. Similarly, one activity in a community sector is not likely to have a widespread effect; for example, implementation of a restrictive worksite policy may push some smokers toward cessation, but more are likely to quit if the policy is accompanied by readily available cessation programs, incentives to achieve cessation, and perhaps a friendly competition to encourage participation. The COMMIT approach includes task forces in at least four key community sectors (described later), involves representatives from diverse community groups, and provides multiple activities in each task force area.

To establish a strong partnership, major components of a community must be involved, not just those groups already concerned with the smoking problem. For a nonsmoking norm to spread to an entire community, representation of the target audience and others not historically involved in tobacco control must be solicited. In addition to spreading the influence of the partnership, such diverse involvement is more likely to have an effect on all of the key groups that are influential in cueing and constraining behavior. Thus, COMMIT sites include representation from the political, economic, religious, education, health, communication, recreational, social, and voluntary associations sectors.

Finally, there must be shared responsibility for the problem, rather than defining it as a problem for a target group alone. It is now clear that smoking affects many people, not merely the person who engages in the behavior. Within the partnership, there must be recognition that all parties must work together and take responsibility for addressing the problem. COMMIT attempts to achieve this by focusing on smoking as a public health issue, rather than a problem for smokers alone; thus, the emphasis is on changing environments and offering smokers repeated opportunities to achieve cessation.

PARTNERSHIP AND TRIAL INTEGRITY

The general principle of "ownership" and its related tenets have been adopted by the COMMIT project. Early in the trial, however, it was recognized that a community organization approach, especially one that emphasizes local control, presented problems for a multi-site study. Total local ownership might result in significantly different organizational structures to accomplish the work of the trial, and thus could compromise the scientific integrity of the trial. Indeed, there was a worry that the project might produce eleven different demonstrations, rather than one trial. On the other hand, too much mandated structure threatens the local ownership of the project, and could negate all of the desirable features of a locally owned and managed project. After much discussion, a compromise approach, designed to achieve trial integrity and still provide enough flexibility to accommodate local variations, was developed.

Trial integrity is achieved in a number of ways. A general mobilization process was followed for organizing the intervention communities. In addition, the trial protocol provides a basic structure for organizing local projects; the required structure was a Community Board and four Task Forces. A set of mandated intervention activities was devised to provide a minimum "dose" of intervention. Lastly, careful documentation of local activities and progress was instituted to monitor compliance with the protocol.

The model developed does not meet all the criteria of an equal partnership with the community [30]. As in other community projects with a research agenda [31, 32], scientific goals in this project are a higher priority than the community development goals [33]. The Research Institutions (RIs), for example, are in charge of administration of the community projects and thereby control budgets, staffing, and the implementation of the protocol. By setting up the RI as the arbiter of compliance with the research aims of the project, lines of authority and responsibility are necessarily established between the partners, with the RI having the authority to negate a decision made by the Community Board. Care was taken, however, to leave decision-making as to how activities and interventions are implemented to the Boards.

MOBILIZATION

The process of initial mobilization of a community group to participate in the COMMIT project was only partially standardized. The first step in mobilization was to understand the community. Prior to randomization, all sites had conducted a community analysis of their sites. The analysis entailed collection of extensive information about the communities, including identification of media outlets, health care providers, worksites, local organizations, available cessation resources, and local schools. The data gathered had both evaluation and intervention purposes. The data provided the bases for sampling frames used for surveying various populations, but were also used to identify groups and individuals who might wish to participate in the project. From that analysis, sites had information on a variety of key sectors and "players" in their communities. The analysis also resulted in an initial description of the community and a crude assessment of potential intervention channels and opportunities.

After randomization, each site conducted a more intensive community analysis to fully understand the intervention community. This involved in-depth examination of the intervention channels to be used in the project as well as an assessment of overall facilitating and inhibiting factors that might affect trial success (see Table 1).

The community analyses also show intervention communities with some variation. There is, as can be seen in Table 2, diversity in the types of communities included; communities vary in terms of size, geographic location, ethnic diversity, and setting.

Three sites, Paterson, Vallejo, and Yonkers, are part of larger urban settings, while others, including the Northwest, mid-American, Canadian, and some of the

Table 2. Characteristics of Intervention Communities

Community	Population (x 1000)	Geographic Location	Percent Ethnic Minority	Setting
Vallejo, CA	89	West	32.7	Urban
Cedar Rapids, IA	145	Midwest	3.7	Self-contained
Fitchburg/Leominster, MA	76	East	4.6	Self-contained
Paterson, NJ	138	East	58.9	Urban
Santa Fe, NM	58	Southwest	37.9	Self-contained
Yonkers, NY	63	East	27.1	Urban
Utica, NY	85	East	7.6	Self-contained
Raleigh, NC	163	South	23.0	Self-contained
Brantford, ON, CAN	87	East	N/A	Self-contained
Medford/Ashland, OR	59	West	5.0	Self-contained
Bellingham, WA	66	West	5.8	Self-contained

Northeast sites are smaller cities that share few services and amenities with other towns (self-contained). Sites also differ in the numbers of smokers and likely access of smokers to intervention channels in the community (see Table 3). The East Coast sites have higher proportions of smokers compared to other sites.

Three communities, Vallejo, Paterson, and Yonkers have relatively low percentages of smokers who work in their communities; similarly, Paterson and Yonkers have lower percentages of smokers who receive health care in the community. In another channel for intervention, public education, all sites are served by media; however, some sites have multiple print and electronic media services, while others share media with the comparison community, making it a difficult channel for intervention.

As part of the community analysis, sites developed a description of the key community sectors whose participation was considered essential, in that community, for the project to proceed. When the community analysis was completed, sites moved to the second step of mobilization, which required activation of a core group of individuals and organizations to work together on the problem. Project staff in each site established a community planning group (CPG). The planning groups consisted of community members who were knowledgeable about the community, who had some commitment to the project, and who were willing to serve for at least a relatively short time on the project. The primary activities to be completed by the CPG were to: 1) provide input into and refinements of the community analysis; 2) develop a plan for forming a more permanent community board (CB); 3) identify and recruit potential CB members; 4) hire a field director to guide the local activities; and 5) develop a plan for establishing and staffing a

Table 3. Number of Smokers and Access to
Selected Intervention Channels by Community

	Percent[a] Smokers	Percent Heavy Smokers	Percent[b] Receiving Health Care in Community	Percent[b] Working in Community	Number of Regional Media Outlets	
					Print	Electronic
Vallejo, CA	28.7	9.4	80.9	46.8	8	21
Cedar Rapids, IA	26.8	11.7	94.4	92.4	2	23
Fitchburg/Leominster, MA	31.3	13.3	84.8	59.1	6	4
Paterson, NJ	31.3	8.8	68.6	40.5	2	13
Santa Fe, NM	23.3	5.1	89.0	85.5	4	47
Yonkers, NY	29.4	10.1	77.7	42.8	4	5
Utica, NY	32.4	12.7	90.2	76.3	1	10
Raleigh, NC	24.9	8.7	88.3	85.7	3	18
Brantford, ON, CAN	35.2	18.6	92.1	84.3	2	51
Medford/Ashland, OR	24.6	8.5	87.1	82.6	5	15
Bellingham, WA	23.9	7.9	90.4	82.2	1	8

[a] Adults aged 25 to 64 years.
[b] Percent of heavy smokers.

local program office. These initial mobilizing activities were to be completed over a very short period of time (approximately five months), that commenced during the summer of 1988. Attainment of those milestones varied by site. All of the sites formed their CPG within three months of randomization of communities to intervention or comparison status; all had field directors by October (five months after randomization), and were in field offices by the end of the year (seven months post-randomization).

The basic organizational structure for the local projects is a broad-based community board with a minimum of four task forces. The task forces correspond to the major intervention channels, and include the Public Education Task Force, oriented to working with the media, promoting community-wide events, and involving youth in tobacco control activities [34]; the Health Care Provider Task Force, responsible for training health care providers to implement regular smoking cessation activities and non-smoking policies in health care settings [35]; the Worksites and Organizations Task Force, responsible for promoting non-smoking policies and providing supportive and promotional activities in worksite and organization settings [36]; and the Cessation Resources and Services Task Force, responsible for enhancing knowledge and awareness of local cessation resources [37]. The four task force areas were selected to provide the broad-based, multi-dimensional approach assumed to be required for successful community change.

The specific task force activities are based on the best available knowledge regarding smoking control; efficacious interventions were extracted from approximately sixty studies commissioned by the National Cancer Institute, as well as community studies in the cardiovascular risk reduction field, and these were the basis for designating the four task force areas.

Once the Community Boards were in place, they were charged with a number of organizational activities, including: 1) definition of the Board mandate; 2) developing by-laws; 3) review/revision of the community analysis; 4) developing a plan to recruit task force members; and 5) development of a plan for local management of the project. Community Board composition and size varied somewhat across sites, although there is great similarity in the types of representatives on the Boards. Most Boards, for example, include health care providers, educators, representatives from local worksites and organizations, union representatives, political figures, and representatives from the major health voluntary groups. Most Boards included some smoker representation.

Community Boards vary in size from twelve to thirty-seven members with the average being nineteen. The time required for recruiting task forces varied from three months to five months, with one site forming both Board and Task Forces simultaneously. All sites had Board by-laws in place by April of 1989, and the majority of sites had a plan for Board management of the field operations (Field Site Management Plan) by that same time.

There was also some diversity in the types of community organizational structures that resulted. Although sites were mandated to form a Community Board and at least four Task Forces, variations were allowed if appropriate for that community. The basic model was followed by all sites, although there was some variation in governance. Some sites added an executive committee to make decisions for the Board. Others relied on Board chairs to make such decisions. Two sites have a broader community coalition or council, in addition to the Board, that meets annually or semi-annually to review project directions and progress. Some sites have added additional Task Forces (e.g., a youth task force, a community outreach task force) to the four mandated ones. These were added because the local Boards believed these areas needed extra or specialized attention to achieve the project goals.

SITE RESPONSES TO PROTOCOL ACTIVITIES

Since sites varied in a number of key facilitators and inhibitors, as well as general sociodemographic characteristics, it was expected that sites would mobilize their communities in different ways and at different speeds. For those communities with considerable experience in developing coalitions, a history of working cooperatively together, and a supportive state or city atmosphere around smoking control, one would expect a faster start in community organization and also community ownership of the project. For sites with less experience working

Table 4. Dates of Attainment of Initial Community Board
Intervention Activities

	Smoking Control Plan	Annual Action Plan 1	Annual Action Plan 2	"Kickoff" Event
Vallejo, CA	5/1[a]	6/8	6/8	7/11
Cedar Rapids, IA	5/1	5/17	5/17	6/15
Fitchburg/Leominster, MA	5/25	6/8	6/8	11/15/88
Paterson, NJ	5/17	[b]	5/17	9/11
Santa Fe, NM	5/1	6/1	6/1	2/21
Yonkers, NY	7/1	7/27	7/27	5/1
Utica, NY	4/13	5/23	5/23	11/10/88
Raleigh, NC	3/16	6/1	6/1	5/1
Brantford, ON, CAN	6/14	5/18	5/18	6/14
Medford/Ashland, OR	3/20	5/31	5/31	2/13
Bellingham, WA	4/21	5/23	5/23	10/4/88

[a] Date notation is mm/dd, where mm is the month and dd is the day, and the year is 1989, unless designated by mm/dd/yy, where yy is the last two digits of the year.
[b] This site did not prepare an Action Plan for the first year.

together, where smoking is not at all a concern, or where other issues dominate the community environment, one would expect a longer mobilization phase as well as a need for more investigator guidance and direction.

The effect of the differences first appeared in movement from the Community Planning Group to the full Community Board. This transition was deliberately left vague because it was expected that communities would vary in their abilities to collaborate in tackling community issues and to form partnerships. In general, transitions occurred when the planning groups felt confident that a sufficient number of people had been recruited to the newly established Community Board. The official transition date varied among sites, as did the number of meetings required before the transition was made. One site, New Mexico, moved almost directly to a Community Board, while most sites required about three months and three to four meetings to make the transition.

Of more interest, perhaps, are the accomplishments of the initial tasks expected to be completed by the Community Board (see Table 4). These planning activities provide the framework on which the four intervention years of the trial are built. The smoking control plan was a community document that outlined the smoking problem in the community and identified the ways in which the local COMMIT project would address that problem. The annual action plans were detailed descriptions of the specific activities to be done, who would do them, when they would be done, and the resources required for conducting the activities. The local project was introduced to the community in a kickoff event that included a news conference and other activities designed to foster awareness of the tobacco problem. There is considerable variety in terms of the amount of time required to meet those objectives. Although "deadlines" were established by the protocol, some sites found it difficult to meet those timelines because of extensive mobilization demands required to recruit and train volunteers to participate in the project. It appears, in general, that larger, more urban, diverse sites require more time for initial mobilization than smaller, more self-contained sites. It may be that the diversity, the greater geographic spread, and competing issues in a large urban setting required more intensive organizational efforts. Other community projects have also noted that more complex environments are more difficult to mobilize [38]. It appears, however, there are enough exceptions among the eleven sites to warrant further study concerning the mobilization timing.

In addition to the differences in time required to complete tasks, there was considerable diversity in the approaches used to achieve them. In some sites, the Community Board and Task Forces did the majority of the work, while others relied more heavily on the research staff. The production of the smoking control plan provides a good example. Sites were to work with their Boards to produce a comprehensive framework for the smoking control activities that would take place over the trial intervention period. In some sites, project staff, by request of the Board, took on the responsibility of preparing that document; in contrast, in some sites the Community Boards wrote the entire document.

The "products" of the sites also varied; for example, some sites elected to produce a slick, smoking control plan to sell the project to the community and others did not. Sites also had to prepare Annual Action Plans that specified, for the first two intervention years, exactly what would be done to meet the trial mandated activities and any other tobacco control activities considered important by the community. In producing the Annual Action Plans, some sites provided detail concerning what groups or individuals were to conduct activities, how much each activity was projected to cost and other information sufficient to guide each and every project activity, while others presented a more general plan that lacked that level of specificity.

The nature of the "partnerships" established between research institutions (RI) and the communities differed between sites. The research requirements of the project meant that communities were not able to make all key decisions regarding the intervention. The ambiguity of the role of the Research Institution relative to that of the Community Board led to some tension, as the lines of authority and responsibility made it clear that the partners were not equal. In some cases, the RI was viewed with suspicion because of its academic focus; local community members were uneasy about being test "subjects" for an experiment. In other sites, the Community Board responded somewhat negatively to the project constraints and proposed tobacco control strategies. Despite these tensions, all sites were able to form an initial partnership between RI and community; however, it appears as though the basis and form of the partnership continues to evolve and will be modified as the trial continues.

DISCUSSION

As COMMIT finished its first intervention year, it was obvious that sites were making good progress in planning for change. All sites had active boards and task forces and had mobilized their communities to address the smoking problem. All sites had produced a comprehensive smoking plan that set out the framework for its activities over the intervention years. All sites had the required task forces and had begun implementing specific interventions. All of these activities put together suggest that the communities have been mobilized and that initial structures are in place to conduct the intervention activities of the trial.

This experience suggests that a structured approach to community mobilization is possible. Eleven quite different communities have followed a protocol to organize their communities around the smoking problem. Although the communities vary, they have formed organizations that meet the requirements of the protocol–that is, a local Board that controls and manages the project–as well as community-specific requirements–for example, the creation of additional task forces. At the same time, communities have been able to take advantage of their own unique characteristics to shape both the organization of the local projects and the implementation of activities.

The structured approach to mobilization is not without its problems. The structural constraints of standardization and contractual obligations resulted in inherent opportunities for tension and the majority of sites did experience some friction in establishing the initial partnership. Because the trial required some standardization, it was difficult to identify the responsibility and authority boundaries of the RI and the Community Boards. According to trial "rules," the RI has the ability to override decisions made by the Board if those decisions threaten the scientific integrity of the trial. In addition, the RI is contractually responsible for the administration of the finances of the site, as well as the actions of paid staff. All of this led to periodic partnership tensions to be expected where one partner clearly has more control over resources than the other. To further exacerbate the situation, the structural constraint of working within a federal contract led to a cumbersome, confusing, and time-consuming budgetary process that frustrated the project staff working in the community. Finally, a protocol that specifies particular activities to be implemented necessarily meant that communities had less than total autonomy over the way smoking control activities were to be developed. For some sites, this resulted in additional tension in building the partnership.

In summary, the use of a standardized community mobilization approach and the inclusion of several principles of community organization into the project was successful in mobilizing communities around the COMMIT project. A major challenge in the remaining years of the COMMIT trial will be to assess whether the differences in the communities, the differences in organizational structures established in the communities, or the resolution of tensions in the partnership will have an effect on the outcome of the trial. The extensive process evaluation incorporated into the COMMIT project will provide useful information about these issues [39]. The experimental design and evaluation plan described elsewhere in this issue [40] will provide rigorous data on trial outcomes. At this point it does appear that, with careful planning, it is possible to develop a protocol for community organization and mobilization that balances the research requirements of a trial with the needs of a community

REFERENCES

1. U.S. Department of Health and Human Services, *Reducing the Health Consequences of Smoking: 25 Years of Progress. A Report of the Surgeon General*, U.S. Department of Health and Human Services, Public Health Service, Centers for Disease Control, Center for Chronic Disease Prevention and Health Promotion, Office on Smoking and Health, DHHS Publication No. (CDC) 89-8411, Prepublication version, 1989.

2. U.S. Department of Health and Human Services, *The Health Consequences of Smoking: Nicotine Addiction. A Report of the Surgeon General*, U.S. Department of Health and Human Services, Public Health Service, Centers for Disease Control, Center for Chronic Disease Prevention and Health Promotion, Office on Smoking and Health, DHHS Publication No. (CDC) 88-8406, 1988.

3. D. C. Iverson, Smoking Control Programs: Premises and Promises, *American Journal of Health Promotion, 1*:3, pp. 16-31, 1987.

4. J. K. Ockene and P. M. Camic, Public Health Approaches to Cigarette Smoking Cessation, *Annuals of Behavioral Medicine, 7*, pp. 14-18, 1985.

5. D. B. Abrams, J. P. Elder, R. A. Carleton, T. M. Lasater, and L. M. Artz, Social Learning Principles for Organizational Health Promotion: An Integrated Approach, in *Health and Industry: A Behavioral Medicine Perspective*, M. F. Cataldo and T. J. Coates (eds.), Wiley-Interscience Publications, New York, 1986.

6. S. J. Feinhandler, The Social Role of Smoking, in *Smoking and Society*, R. D. Tollinson (ed.), Lexington Books, Lexington, Massachusetts, 1986.

7. A. McAlister, P. Puska, J. T. Salonen, J. Toumilehto, and K. Koskela, Theory and Action for Health Promotion: Illustrations from the North Karelia Project, *American Journal of Public Health, 72*, pp. 43-50, 1982.

8. S. Sussman, Two Social Influence Perspectives of Tobacco Use Development and Prevention, *Health Education Research, 4*:2, pp. 213-223, 1989.

9. N. Maccoby, The Community as a Focus for Health Promotion, in *The Social Psychology of Health*, S. Spacapan and S. Oskamp (eds.), Sage Publications, Newberry Park, California, 1988.

10. G. S. Omenn, B. Thompson, M. Sexton, N. Hessol, B. Breitenstein, S. Curry, M. Michnick, and A. Peterson, A Randomized Comparison of Worksite-Sponsored Smoking Cessation Programs, *American Journal of Prevention Medicine, 4*:5, pp. 261-267, 1988.

11. W. J. Millar and B. E. Naegele, Time to Quit: Community Involvement in Smoking Cessation, *Canadian Journal of Public Health, 78*, pp. 109-114, 1987.

12. A. Wandersman and P. Florin, An Introduction to Citizen Participation, Voluntary Organizations and Community Development: Insights for Empowerment through Research, *American Journal of Community Psychology*, 1989.

13. A. Englund, Strategies for Prevention: Role of Voluntary and Community Organizations in Implementation, *Cancer Detection and Prevention, 9*, pp. 413-415, 1986.

14. L. Wallack, A Community Approach to the Prevention of Alcohol-Related Problems: The San Francisco Experience, *International Quarterly of Community Health Education, 5*:2, pp. 85-102, 1985.

15. L. Wallack and D. Barrows, *Preventing Alcohol Problems in California: Evaluation of the Three Year "Winners" Program*, California Department of Alcohol and Drug Programs, Sacramento, California, 1981.

16. J. M. Raeburn and F. W. Seymour, A Simple Systems Model for Community Programs, *Journal of Community Psychology, 7*, pp. 290-297, 1979.

17. A. J. Stunkard, M. R. J. Felix, and R. Y. Cohen, Mobilizing a Community to Promote Health, in *Prevention in Health Psychology*, J. C. Rosen and L. J. Solomon (eds.), University Press of New England, Hanover, New Hampshire, 1985.

18. I. Robertson, *Sociology*, Worth Publishers, New York, 1977.

19. M. Pertschuk and D. R. Shopland, *Major Local Smoking Ordinances in the United States*, U.S. Department of Health and Human Services, Public Health Service, National Institute of Health, National Cancer Institute, NIH Publication No. 90-479, September, 1989.

20. K. E. Warner, Smoking and Health Implications of a Change in the Federal Cigarette Excise Tax, *Journal of the American Medical Association, 255*:8, pp. 1028-1032, February 28, 1986.

21. E. M. Lewit and D. Coate, The Potential for Using Excise Taxes to Reduce Smoking, *Journal of Health Economics, 1*:2, pp. 121-145, 1982.

22. J. Farquhar, The Community-Based Model of Life Style Intervention Trials, *American Journal of Epidemiology, 108*, pp. 103-111, 1978.

23. J. G. Kelly, Tain't What You Do, It's the Way You Do It, *American Journal of Community Psychology, 7*, pp. 239-261, 1979.

24. H. Blackburn, Research and Demonstration Projects in Community Cardiovascular Disease Prevention, *Journal of Public Health Policy, 4*, pp. 398-421, 1983.

25. L. W. Green, The Theory of Participation: A Qualitative Analysis of Its Expression in National and International Health Politics, *Advances in Health Education and Promotion: Vol. 1*, JAI Press, Greenwich, Connecticut, 1986.

26. K. Kurji, T. Ostbye, and T. Bhatti, Initiating Community Self-Help: A Model for Public Health Workers, *Canadian Journal of Public Health, 79*, pp. 208-209, 1988.

27. R. Labonte, Community Empowerment: The Need for Political Analysis, *Canadian Journal of Public Health, 80*, pp. 87-91, 1989.

28. N. Crosby, J. M. Kelly, and P. Schaefer, Citizen Panels: A New Approach to Citizen Participation, *Public Administration Review, 46*:2, pp. 170-178, 1986.

29. L. C. Garro, J. Roulette, and R. G. Whitmore, Community Control of Health Care Delivery: The Sandy Bay Experience, *Canadian Journal of Public Health, 77*, pp. 281-284, 1986.

30. R. F. Allen and J. Allen, A Sense of Community, a Shared Vision and a Positive Culture: Core Enabling Factors in Successful Culture Based Health Promotion, *American Journal of Health Promotion, 1*:3, pp. 40-47, 1987.
31. R. M. Goodman and A. Steckler, A Model for the Institutionalization of Health Promotion Programs, *Community Health, 11*:4, pp. 63-78, 1989.
32. D. M. Chavis, P. E. Stucky, and A. Wandersman, Returning Basic Research to the Community: A Relationship between Scientist and Citizen, *American Psychologist, 36*:4, pp. 424-434, 1983.
33. J. Rothman, Three Models of Community Organization Practice, in *Strategies of Community Organization*, F. M. Cox, J. L. Erlich, J. Rothman, and R. E. Tropman (eds.), Peacock, Itasca, Illinois, 1979.
34. L. Wallack and R. Sciandra, Media Advocacy and Public Education in the Community Intervention Trial to Reduce Heavy Smoking (COMMIT), *International Quarterly of Community Health Education, 11*:3, pp. 205-222, 1990-91.
35. J. K. Ockene, E. L. Lindsay, L. Berger, and N. Hymowitz, Health Care Providers as Key Change Agents in the Community Intervention Trial for Smoking Cessation (COMMIT), *International Quarterly of Community Health, 11*:3, pp. 223-237 1990-91.
36. G. Sorensen, R. E. Glasgow, and K. Corbett, Promoting Smoking Control through Worksites in the Community Intervention Trial for Smoking Cessation (COMMIT), *International Quarterly of Community Health Education,11*:3, pp. 239-257, 1990-91.
37. P. Pomrehn, R. Sciandra, R. Shipley, W. Lynn, and H. Lando, Enhancing Resources for Smoking Cessation through Community Intervention: COMMIT as a Prototype, *International Quarterly of Community Health Education, 11*:3, pp. 259-269, 1990-91.
38. R. A. Smith, Community Structural Characteristics and the Adoption of Fluoridation, *American Journal of Public Health, 71*, pp. 24-30, 1981.
39. K. Corbett, B. Thompson, N. White, and M. Taylor, Process Evaluation in the Community Intervention Trial for Smoking Cessation (COMMIT), *International Quarterly of Community Health Education, 11*:3, pp. 291-309, 1990-91.
40. M. E. Mattson, K. M. Cummings, W. R. Lynn, C. Giffen, D. Corle, and T. Pechacek, Evaluation Plan for the Community Intervention Trial for Smoking Cessation (COMMIT), *International Quarterly of Community Health Education, 11*:3, pp. 271-290, 1990-91.

Direct reprint requests to:

Beti Thompson, Ph.D.
Fred Hutchinson Cancer Research Center
1124 Columbia Street, MP 702
Seattle, WA 98104-2092

MEDIA ADVOCACY AND PUBLIC EDUCATION IN THE COMMUNITY INTERVENTION TRIAL TO REDUCE HEAVY SMOKING (COMMIT)

LAWRENCE WALLACK, DR.PH.
University of California, Berkeley

RUSSELL SCIANDRA, M.A.
Roswell Park Cancer Institute, Buffalo, New York

For the COMMIT Research Group

ABSTRACT

The Community Intervention Trial (COMMIT) is designed to reduce the rate of heavy smoking in eleven pairs of North American communities over an eight-year period. The intervention, consisting of a minimum of fifty-one activities, is being implemented through local community boards and task forces. This article describes the goals and activities for the public education task force with a specific focus on "media advocacy," an innovative use of mass media that follows more closely political activist models than traditional public service models. Two brief case studies are presented to illustrate some applications of media advocacy. The reasons for relatively infrequent use of media advocacy are discussed.

The use of tobacco is a problem of enormous public health significance. In the United States almost 50 million people continue to smoke cigarettes and approximately 390,000 deaths are linked to cigarette smoking each year [1]. The cost to the nation in terms of health expenses and lost time from work totals $52 billion or approximately $221 per person [2]. Worldwide, annually 2.5 million deaths are linked to tobacco use and the toll is likely to increase. Cigarette smoking has been called the "emerging epidemic" in developing countries [3, 4]. In China, for

Int'l. Quarterly of Community Health Education, Vol. 11(3) 205-222, 1990-91

© 1991, Baywood Publishing Co., Inc.

example, it is estimated that 50 million of the current population of children will eventually die of tobacco related illness [5].

The *Community Intervention Trial* for Smoking Cessation (COMMIT) represents the most comprehensive planning, implementation and evaluation effort to reduce smoking through community approaches attempted to date. COMMIT, funded by the National Cancer Institute, extends over an eight-year period and involves eleven pairs of communities randomized within pairs to intervention or comparison status. An extensive process and outcome evaluation is integrated into the overall project and is reviewed elsewhere in this journal [6, 7].

The overall goal of COMMIT is to reduce the number of heavy smokers (25+ cigarettes daily). There are fifty-one required smoking control activities which make up the COMMIT protocol. These activities are implemented in each intervention site stressing community mobilization and development of a board comprised of a diverse group of community representatives [8-11].

The purpose of this article is to review the use of mass media as a strategy for public education in the COMMIT sites. Specific attention will be provided to the use of "media advocacy" which has been developed for the COMMIT project. Media advocacy differs from the usual public relations type of activity and attempts to focus on the social and political aspects of tobacco control issues.

MASS MEDIA AND SMOKING CONTROL AT THE COMMUNITY LEVEL

The mass media serve in some ways to facilitate smoking control efforts and in other ways to inhibit these efforts. The inhibiting role can be seen in three specific areas. First, cigarette advertisements communicate inaccurate information by linking the product with images of health, fitness, beauty and social acceptance [12]. Second, it is becoming increasingly apparent that cigarette advertising results in increased consumption [13, 14]. Third, the economic influence of tobacco advertising results in limited coverage of the adverse health effects of cigarettes. This self-censorship has been well documented with regard to magazines where articles detailing the health consequences associated with smoking are absent or extremely infrequent [15, 16]. For example, the significant news that lung cancer had replaced breast cancer as the leading cause of cancer death among women was remarkably ignored in the pages of many women's magazines [17].

On the other hand, the mass media represent an important resource for community interventions attempting to reduce premature death and disability associated with cigarette smoking. The mass media contribute significantly to the overall context in which personal decisions about initiating, continuing, or quitting smoking occur. Further, the media are a key source of social-environmental cues regarding non-smoking behavior. In addition, the public health-oriented framing of tobacco issues in the mass media can contribute to popular support for smoke-free policies and make it easier for legislators and other politicians to provide their support.

Historically, the mass media have played a number of important roles in smoking prevention and control. These include informing the public about the hazards of smoking, contributing to norms that reinforce non-smoking behavior, directly encouraging smoking cessation attempts, and, more lately, trying to strip the tobacco industry of its legitimacy.

Warner used econometric analysis to estimate the effect of publicity regarding the hazards of smoking from the early 1960s to the mid-1970s [18]. He found a significant cumulative effect of the publication of the 1964 Surgeon General's Report, the radio and television broadcast of anti-smoking ads from 1968-1970 resulting from the application of the Fairness Doctrine, and continuing publicity through the 1970s. Specifically, he estimated that per capita consumption of cigarettes would have been one-fifth to one-third greater had there been no anti-smoking publicity.

In a review of fifty-six evaluated mass media programs to reduce cigarette smoking among adults, Flay found that these programs achieved a number of objectives [19]. These included success in informing and motivating people to quit; getting potential quitters to take a specific action such as calling a hotline number or quitting for a day; and, getting smokers to quit over an extended period. For example, a one year follow-up of a televised smoking cessation program aired in connection with a self-help program reported 25 percent of study participants were not smoking and 10 percent had been continuously smoke free [20]. While fewer than 500 people had requested self-help manuals in previous years, 50,000 people obtained manuals in conjunction with the televised program. Even with lower quit rates than occur in group and clinic settings (which was not the case in this study) the substantially larger number of people exposed to the intervention ultimately results in greater numbers of people attempting to quit and maintaining smoke-free lives.

Cummings et al., reported that a smoking cessation series in a Buffalo, New York newspaper induced more than 9600 smokers to quit smoking for at least one week. This represented 4 percent of the smokers in the target population [21].

In Australia a mass media campaign using paid placements for advertisements emphasizing the health consequences of smoking was found to result in a short (6 months) and long-term (3 year) reduction in smoking prevalence, though primarily for men. This campaign was linked to activities at the school, organizational and general community level [22].

The use of media to recruit smokers into cessation programs has also shown some promising results. A randomized community trial of a media campaign recruiting young women smokers to call a cessation hotline showed a ten-fold increase in calls from intervention television markets when compared to the control markets. Those groups which were specifically targeted showed an increase of twenty-fold. Nearly 50 percent of calls received during the seven-month campaign occurred during a three week period in which television time was purchased [23].

Most recently smoking control advocates have taken an aggressive approach to using mass media. This "media advocacy" approach is illustrated in the careful negative framing by anti-smoking advocates of RJR-Nabisco efforts to target women (Dakota brand) and minorities (Uptown brand) with new brands of cigarettes [24, 25]. In addition, the activities of local groups around the country who are protesting the use of billboards to advertise cigarettes and alcohol in minority communities reflects a media advocacy approach [26-28].

Community-wide smoking interventions are based on an important assumption that many of the key circumstances supporting both smoking and the decision to quit are social and not just individual circumstances. Intervention strategies, rather than targeting individuals, aim at generating group influence and social support directed toward smoking cessation. Important elements of the individual's social network, such as the worksite and health care providers, have been identified as key points at which such influences can be applied.

Media differs from other elements of the social network in that it is largely through the media that individuals form their perception of community-wide beliefs with regard to smoking. In addition to providing information about smoking to large numbers of people over a short span of time, the mass media can directly affect community norms. Mass media functions in three ways that influence the climate of public attitudes.

First, mass media is often able to set the public agenda. It is often said that the media may not tell people what to think but do tell people what to think about. Second, the media confer status and legitimacy on various topics or points of view which are selected out for attention. The presence of a topic in the media helps to establish its importance. Third, the mass media can activate and stimulate public discussion. It also provides the framework for the discussion by roughly establishing the boundaries of legitimate discourse.

Public Education Goals for COMMIT

The overall strategy for public education strategies in COMMIT is to stimulate public debate about smoking to help create a community environment in which the benefits of non-smoking are widely accepted and the advantages and opportunities for cessation are widely known. Such an environment, it is thought, serves to increase sentiment favoring public policy initiatives and expansion of community resources for tobacco control. At the same time, social support for continued smoking is eroded.

Three goals guide the use of mass media for public education in COMMIT:

1. promote social norms and actions toward a smoke-free community.
2. promote the importance of smoking as a public health issue; and,
3. enhance the effectiveness of smoking control in other program areas.

- Increase the percentage of people identifying smoking as a serious public health issue to 75%;

- Increase the percentage of people perceiving strong community norms supporting a smoke-free environment to 60%;

- Increase the percentage of heavy smokers who attempt to quit during the Great American Smokeout (an annual event sponsored by the American Cancer Society) to 35%; and,

- Increase the percentage of non-smokers who participate in smoking control activities to 12%.

Figure 1. Impact objectives for 1993 (end of trial).

Inherent in these goals is the use of media in conjunction with, rather than instead of or apart from, a range of smoking control and cessation activities. Progress toward these goals will be assessed by tracking a series of impact and process objectives [6, 7]. The impact objectives are shown in Figure 1. To achieve these objectives six protocol activities are mandated (see Figure 2). Each activity is described in the protocol. The resources needed to accomplish the activity are listed and those responsible for implementing the activity are noted. In addition, each activity includes quantifiable process objectives which are tracked. These activities can be divided into three main areas: those aimed at increasing visibility of and support for COMMIT; those which promote individual attempts to quit smoking; and, those which enhance news coverage of smoking issues, seeking to reframe the terms of public debate.

Two protocol activities are primarily concerned with establishing and maintaining the visibility and credibility of COMMIT in the community. The program has been introduced to each intervention community at a required kickoff news event which included appropriate influentials from local government and organizations. Later, the strategic Smoking Control Plan was unveiled at a press conference, and each year the Annual Action Plan is publicized with a similar event. A trial-wide publicity resource kit has been distributed to each site to assist in the implementation of these activities, but each has retained a local character suitable to the community.

An important aspect of these activities is that they serve not only to heighten awareness of COMMIT in the community, but help to frame smoking as an important public health issue in terms which will garner support for the intervention. They are a high visibility forum in which tobacco is presented as a community-wide problem requiring community-wide solutions. The repeated and

• Media Advocacy Training of Board
• Implement Kick-Off Event
• Publicize Smoking Control and Annual Action Plans
• Establish a Community Network to Enhance Local Coverage of National and Regional News
• Design and Implement Magnet Events
• Publicize Smoking Control Activities in Other Task Force Areas

Figure 2. Mandated public education activities.

extensive media coverage which can be attracted helps establish smoking as an important priority on the public agenda.

Two mandated activities and three optional activities are more concerned with promoting cessation directly. Each site is required to implement two magnet events per year. A magnet event is defined as a well publicized, temporally limited activity or set of activities which stimulate smokers to quit and provides opportunities to do so. The best known example of such an event is the American Cancer Society's Great American Smokeout (GASO) and "Weedless Wednesday" which falls in the middle of Non Smoking Week in Canada. In addition to GASO and Non-dependence Day, sponsored by the American Lung Association, sites have initiated other magnet events, most notably community wide "Quit and Win" contests.

Another mandated activity is the use of media to publicize smoking control activities in other intervention channels such as worksites and health care settings. For example, a required, "Ask your physician about smoking" activity is coordinated between the health care and public education task forces. In addition, each site is required to develop and implement annual media plans for advertising the availability of services such as a smokers' hotline and a cessation resources directory. Broadcast media, newspapers, billboards, posters and pamphlets may all be part of these campaigns, with the allocation of resources varying widely depending on the circumstances in each community.

There are a number of optional activities that sites can do after the required activities have been conducted. Sites may elect to develop a mass media education or cessation campaign using purchased or donated time and space. The intensity of such campaigns would vary widely across the sites depending on the availability of local resources, use of paid media and the priority of the activity for the local group. However, it is anticipated that existing materials will be adapted to local needs to minimize production costs.

The use of paid media is allowed if the task force makes it a line item in the budget and it is approved by the Community Board. Some sites have been successful in leveraging matching public service time or space in exchange for paid advertising.

THE BASICS OF MEDIA ADVOCACY

Media advocacy has been developed for COMMIT sites as an innovative approach to the use of media for smoking control. "Media advocacy," according to Michael Pertschuk one of the architects of this approach, "is the strategic use of mass media for advancing a social or public policy initiative" [29]. Media advocacy promotes a range of strategies to stimulate broad-based media coverage to reframe public debate to increase public support for more effective policy level approaches to public health problems. It does not attempt to directly change individual risk behavior but focuses attention on changing the way the problem is understood as a public health issue. For example, a media advocacy approach might develop a strategy to stimulate media coverage regarding the ethical and legal culpability of tobacco companies that promote deadly products to teenagers. The purpose is to shift attention from defining smoking solely as an individual problem and highlight the role of those who shape the environment in which individual decisions about health-related behavior are made.

All media coverage of health, whether news, entertainment or public service, will tend to increase awareness and knowledge regarding health issues. Social marketing, social advertising (e.g., Partnership for a Drug Free America) and public communication campaigns in general serve this purpose. The essence of media advocacy, however, is to move beyond this function and involve the public in the policy generating process [30]. The goal is to empower the public to more fully participate in defining the social and political environment in which decisions affecting health are made.

Media advocacy is issue oriented. It recognizes that the mass media are often the forum for contesting major policies that affect health. Unfortunately the public debate tends to be narrowly defined by ideological (individual-focused explanations) and practical (limited time to present complex issues) considerations of media coverage, and the concerns of vested interest groups. Overcoming these barriers represents a major challenge for media advocacy.

There are a number of skills that are key for the media advocate. These include research, "creative epidemiology," issue framing, and gaining access to media outlets. Research is important in becoming a reliable and credible media advocate. The advocate must not only know the key studies, significant data, and contested issues regarding the particular topic, but must also know the characteristics of the various media outlets. For example, the anti-smoking activist might regularly screen the local newspaper to identify which reporters cover relevant issues or if the paper has taken editorial positions on related issues.

Creative epidemiology is the use of research and existing data to gain media attention and clearly convey the public health importance of an issue. It *does not* imply a loose use of data or misleading presentation of the facts. On the contrary, because creative epidemiology will stimulate media coverage and, perhaps, generate controversy, it must be scientifically sound. For example, an American Cancer Society videotape explains that, "1000 people quit smoking every day–by dying. That is equivalent to two fully loaded jumbo jets crashing every day, with no survivors." Creative epidemiology frames data to be interesting for the media and more understandable and meaningful to the general public.

Framing the issue to be consistent with policy goals is a complex and sophisticated endeavor. The corporate world is very skilled at using valued symbols to their advantage. For example, legitimate criticism of the marketing practices of tobacco and alcohol producers becomes an "attempt at censorship" or an "assault on the First Amendment." In the United States the corporate world provides funds for local community groups thus buying friends and goodwill. In addition, substantial support is provided to arts and cultural events to purchase "innocence by association" [29]. The industry uses a range of strategies to capture symbols such as freedom of choice, freedom of speech, patron of the arts and many others to stake out the moral high ground and gain widespread support.

Successful framing of an issue puts the media advocate in a more advantageous position. The advocate can determine, to a great extent, the terms of discussion. The tobacco industry has carefully crafted an image of themselves as advocates of civil rights, protector of free speech and good community citizens. Anti-smoking groups were successfully characterized as zealots, health nuts, and health facists. The industry was very successful at this until recently when anti-smoking activists reframed the issues by stripping the industry of its positive symbols. Tobacco producers became "merchants of death," "hitman in three-piece suits," and exploiters of youth, women, and minority groups. A number of strategies were developed to expose and publicize tobacco industry ties to cultural events, "shaming" through public exposure those who accept industry money, and continually making explicit the link between death and tobacco.

Successful reframing uses two primary strategies. First, it focuses attention on industry practices as the primary problem rather than the behavior of the individual. Second, it seeks to delegitimize the industry by exposing industry practices that are exploitive and unethical. Advertising and marketing practices which exploit children and place profits before health and safety provide raw material for the media advocate. This further erodes public support for the particular industry and makes it more difficult to purchase goodwill.

Gaining access to the mass media is fundamental to media advocacy. Historically health educators have been heavily dependent on the willingness of the media to provide time or space. In a sense, the media were allowed to define which issues would be aired and how the discussion would be structured. The availability of public service time is declining as media outlets increase efforts to sell all available time in response to pressures to enhance the "bottom line" [31]. Using creative epidemiology and framing strategies it is possible to have greater control over how the media cover an issue. To be effective it is necessary to take advantage of both free and carefully placed paid media.

It is useful to rethink the concepts of free and paid media. This usually is interpreted to mean the difference between a public service announcement which might air at any time of the day or night or a purchased spot where you can assure desired audience exposure to your spot. In reality there is a wide assortment of good free time for the media advocate to use. The media advocate can *create news* in a number of ways. It is possible to build on to breaking news stories. For example, by creating "local reaction" many communities mobilized media coverage around the release of the Surgeon General's 25th anniversary report on smoking and health. The media advocate also can create news by presenting small research studies of local or national interest. For example, the Center for Science in the Public Interest, a consumer advocacy group, drew attention to the issue of alcohol advertising and children by doing a small study that showed that kids could name more brands of beer than presidents of the United States. This received national attention. The media advocate can build on related news opportunities. For example, when tons of Chilean fruit were banned because of a small amount of cyanide, local anti-smoking activists used this to point out to the media that it would take bushels of grapes to equal the cyanide in the sidestream smoke of just one cigarette.

There are numerous ways that the media advocate can increase coverage of an issue. News coverage can be extended by providing op-ed pieces to newspapers and stimulating letters to the editor. In addition, relationships with print and electronic journalists can be cultivated so that access is gained for follow-up stories with local perspectives. Cultivating access needs to be viewed as a long term, cumulative strategy that will improve with every successful effort.

Media advocacy has several limitations. First, this approach has not been adequately defined and no clear set of principles have been developed. It is an evolving approach that has emerged from grassroots and public interest groups. Second, the skills involved in media advocacy are complex. The media advocate needs to understand the media culture including what is news and how it can be framed to gain media interest and citizen support. Third, the necessary time for research and cultivating media gatekeepers may be beyond the bounds of those working in public agencies. Fourth, media advocacy is linked to an environmental approach that focuses primarily on the social and political aspects of health and is less concerned with direct behavioral change. This focus makes it difficult to get and hold media attention which tends to highlight the personal and individual aspects of health problems. Finally, media advocacy approaches will tend to be controversial because they directly confront powerful vested interests. Health agencies, as well as the media, may be hesitant to work with some advocates on some issues.

MEDIA TRAINING IN COMMIT

The 11 COMMIT sites present a diversity of media environments. Four sites are freestanding media markets, each with at least four broadcast television stations, a dominant local daily newspaper, and a number of radio stations. The other seven sites are part of larger metropolitan markets, with most television stations and the dominant daily newspaper originating outside the intervention community. In two of these sites, the intervention communities share with the comparison communities dominant daily newspapers and at least some of the broadcast outlets. This posed the problem of potential contamination of the comparison community and required careful, very limited use of overlapping media.

Public education through the mass media is an important element of the COMMIT intervention. To insure optimal use of mass media a training was developed for all COMMIT field directors. This training was provided as part of a two day training in the Washington, D.C. area that was held shortly after each site hired a field director. In addition to this central training, several sites have held trainings at the local level to meet the protocol requirement that board members and other intervention staff be trained in a range of mass media techniques. The central media training included a number of topics:

- Building a press strategy
- Identifying and training spokespeople
- Media resource analysis
- Elements of smoking prevention and cessation campaign design
- Strategies for countering tobacco industry promotions; and
- Use of role models.

The media advocacy part of the training was conducted by the Advocacy Institute, an organization specializing in public interest issues with a strong focus on anti-smoking. Specific exercises were used to develop strategies to enhance access to the media, develop overall strategy, and frame issues. Small groups, for example, were given a problem such as the construction of a Camel billboard next to a local high school and asked to develop approaches to get media attention. In addition, strategies for countering tobacco industry arguments were developed in a "Meet the Press" type of format. Finally, guidelines for cultivating and maintaining relationships with the press were presented and discussed. Various written materials were distributed for the field directors to take back to their sites.

MEDIA ACTIVITY IN COMMIT SITES

In general, COMMIT sites have implemented a wide range of media-related activities during the first year of the intervention. Many of these activities have focussed on developing a foundation for future activities by increasing public support and awareness for COMMIT. Sites were successful in gaining publicity for the "kick off" of the project and publicizing the "Smoking Control Plan." Several sites have invited nationally known anti-smoking activists into the community as a way of generating interest and getting media attention. Press conferences, letters to the editor, guest newspaper editorials, and appearances on public affairs programs have been used by various sites.

One of the key resources available to each site is an electronic bulletin board which provides daily summaries of tobacco related stories in major newspapers and periodic action alerts. These alerts provide instant and sometimes advance notice of key smoking stories such as the release of new scientific studies. Along with basic information on the story the alert includes key quotes from major figures, suggestions for framing the story, and suggested "media bites."

Sites, as required by the protocol, have tried to develop local angles on national or regional stories. For example, in some sites interviews with local physicians were arranged to draw attention to new research findings regarding women and smoking.

Several sites have routinely made use of COMMIT survey data in news stories. For example, the headline in one newspaper from the Massachusetts site read, "Poll: Non-smokers back limits." This story reported smokers' responses regarding public policy alternatives to limit smoking in worksites and health facilities and restricting sales to minors. A review of COMMIT activities over the year was also included. Three sites presented data showing support for smoking restrictions and three demonstrated wide backing for actions restricting youth access to tobacco. Four sites used press releases to present statistics on Great American Smokeout participation and provided advertising for the event.

Overall, the kind of media activities commonly conducted by COMMIT serve several purposes. These activities potentially raise public awareness about the risks of smoking, erode public support for tobacco use, and build community support for COMMIT and its basic approach to smoking as a public health problem. Many other activities have more specifically targeted individual smoking and have directly supported cessation activities.

This latter group of activities includes special events such as community-wide "Quit and Win" contests in North Carolina, Canada, Oregon, Utica and Massachusetts, and support for GASO in all U.S. sites. In some sites, paid advertising was used in addition to public service ads and news events to heighten public awareness. In Utica, COMMIT efforts resulted in the local newspaper running a six day series on quitting smoking in the "Lifestyles" section. In the Washington site paid advertising promoted the availability during the Christmas season of a free "Holiday Quit Kit."

Some sites (Utica and Iowa) have initiated paid public awareness campaigns using both locally produced materials and items produced elsewhere and obtained at low cost. Purchasing advertising allows higher visibility and better targeting of messages, while public service advertising often results in limited exposure at best. Media used have included radio, television, print and outdoor. Sites have negotiated with broadcasters to received matching public service spots for each paid ad. In at least two sites, the resources devoted to media production and placement during Year 2 of the intervention were substantial–accounting for approximately 20 percent of implementation funds.

PUBLIC EDUCATION: TWO CASE STUDIES

Oregon

The Oregon COMMIT intervention site involves the neighboring cities of Medford and Ashland, with a combined population of 60,000. The community has three local television stations, ten radio stations, and two daily newspapers. The field director previously worked as the public relations person for a local hospital and came to the project with excellent media contacts and well developed skills.

The field director was trained in media advocacy in October 1988 with the other newly hired field directors. She made use of her media contacts and organized a COMMIT preliminary "kick off" in January to coincide with the release of the 25th Surgeon General's report on smoking and health. The event included the gift of a silver wrapped report to each mayor by the directors of two of the local voluntaries. The headlines from the two local papers captures the dual purpose of the media event: "Anti-smoking campaign gets under way today" and "Ceremony in Ashland marks 25 years of anti-smoking effort." The primary "kick-off" (a required protocol activity), combined with an open house at the COMMIT office, occurred the following month and received newspaper and radio coverage.

In July, a press conference was called after a board meeting to announce the "Annual Action Plan" and "Smoking Control Plan." Press packets were sent out and phone calls were made to insure press attendance. Turnout was excellent and generated the desired coverage. Print stories included quotes from board members, COMMIT staff, some survey data, and a review of the four year plan.

The field director developed a process for working with action alerts and meeting the protocol requirement of developing news releases on the local aspects of national stories. A three-person subcommittee of the Public Education Task Force was formed to discuss which media alerts to act on. For example, in March 1989 it was decided to use the cyanide tainted Chilean grape story to get local attention. The stories offered clear comparisons of the amounts of cyanide in the two products: "A pack a day smoker would have to eat about 3,000 grapes to equal the amount of cyanide he's consuming from cigarettes" and "if the FDA were to take the same action against cigarettes that it has taken against grapes, there would be no cigarettes for sale in this country."

In December 1989 a media advocacy training was conducted locally for board and task force members and COMMIT staff. Fifteen people attended and a new Media Advocacy Subcommittee was formed. Shortly thereafter Philip Morris started their campaign to sponsor the Bill of Rights and the date for all domestic flights to go smoke-free was fast approaching. Both these stories had been followed closely through action alerts. The subcommittee instructed COMMIT staff to approach the editor of the largest newspaper to write an editorial against the Philip Morris campaign. The editor stated his opposed viewpoint to the COMMIT staff who offered no counter argument but, as they anticipated, he offered them space for a guest editorial. An editorial was drafted by the Board Chair (a smoker), revised to exclude a final paragraph which might have been construed as lobbying (an activity prohibited because of COMMIT's federal funding) and was approved by the full Board. Eventually, the guest editorial was run in both local papers.

To draw attention to the smoking ban on domestic flights a press conference was held at the local airport on the first day of the ban. The Board Chair and the Director of the County Health and Human Services Department attended along with twenty children from the Smoke Free American project. They met an incoming flight and passed out Lung Association "Survival Kits" to those sitting in the smoking section of the airport. All three local television stations attended.

The Oregon site appears to have cultivated excellent relations with local media. COMMIT press events are well attended by the media who respond to press releases and telephone calls. Television and newspapers routinely appear but radio stations have less frequently attended. The field director reports that they sometimes receive calls from newspapers to get updates on COMMIT progress.

One of the potential problems of having a focus on local media (the protocol requires at least eight press releases on local angles of major national stories each year) is that there is too much smoking news and media outlets get overwhelmed. To protect against burnout the Oregon site rotates coverage of COMMIT activities across the three television stations. For example, one station will be provided with background for a story and access to key people as an exclusive. Another potential problem is that local media might feel manipulated when sites attempt to sensationalize stories to point out the risk of smoking. After working on the Chilean grape story the Oregon site decided to forego a related story on the health risks of contaminated Perrier water versus that of cigarettes. It was felt that local media might not respond well to this topic.

Utica

Utica, population 86,000, is located in a largely rural area of upstate New York. Utica has two local television stations, fourteen radio stations and one local newspaper. The Field Director came to the project with little prior media experience but has been very active in this area.

In December 1989, Utica COMMIT conducted a media advocacy training program which was attended by fifteen task force members and community agency representatives. An important aspect of the program was exercises to stimulate new, creative approaches to gaining access to the media.

A primary strategy in Utica has been to portray the tobacco industry as the opponent of community health. Recruiting a variety of local spokespersons to represent COMMIT has reinforced its image as a community-based organization in opposition to the industry outsider. In addition to focusing attention of the industry rather than individual smokers as the "enemy," this strategy has the added benefit of framing smoking and health issues in terms of conflict, which appeal to an important media gatekeeper criterion for newsworthiness. When possible, press releases confront the tobacco industry as "merchants of death" and an unethical corporate citizen.

Several events have been designed to specifically focus on tobacco industry marketing techniques. On separate occasions two national figures, Alan Blum, M.D., founder of Doctors Ought to Care (DOC), and David Goerlitz, a former cigarette advertising model, were brought to the community to make presentations and stimulate media coverage. In another instance, the U.S. Boomerang Team which had refused sponsorship by Philip Morris performed an exhibition at a local minor league baseball game and met with the media about the issue of tobacco sports sponsorship.

In March 1989, COMMIT took advantage of the nomination of William Bennett, at that time a heavy smoker, as Drug Czar. It organized a news conference at which the COMMIT field director, executive director of the Council on Alcoholism, and director of a drug treatment center praised Bennett for setting a good example by quitting cigarettes and called for a comprehensive campaign against all drugs, including tobacco.

Another example of media advocacy occurred in reaction to the appearance in the community of a national dance company sponsored by Philip Morris. On the night of the performance COMMIT volunteers stood in front of the theater distributing handbills. A news release resulted in substantial newspaper and television coverage of the demonstration which featured a locally prominent chest surgeon saying that he was distributing the handbills, "because cigarettes are killing people."

The text of the handbill depicted Philip Morris as a "merchant of death" seeking to buy respectability through its support for the dance company. A chart presented disease-specific mortality attributable to Philip Morris products based on the company's share of total cigarette sales. This creative presentation of the data powerfully conveyed the message of health hazards of smoking to the individual, at the same time identifying the cigarette industry rather than its victims as the source of the problem.

Through this event Utica smokers were exposed to news accounts in which a doctor called cigarette advertising lies and said that not smoking is the only protection against lung disease. While this information may be no different from that presented in a typical public service announcement, COMMIT, using media advocacy techniques, was able to present it in a different format (television news and newspaper entertainment review), reach a wide audience with a credible spokesperson (chest surgeon), and create a dramatic context in which to convey the information.

Utica COMMIT has worked hard to cultivate positive relationships with the news media and is seen as a credible, reliable source of newsworthy stories. Television, newspaper, and radio stations with news department regularly cover COMMIT-initiated events and press conferences. This interest has extended to public affairs programming and newspaper feature departments, which have been responsive to COMMIT proposals.

DISCUSSION

Media advocacy approaches have been used by the sites in a limited way. For example, all sites appear to benefit from the action alerts and gain considerable information about key public policy issues. These action alerts have been used extensively to meet protocol requirements. To some extent the framing issues and creative epidemiology aspects of media advocacy have had much more limited use. The least used advocacy strategies have been the ones which tend to be the most confrontational. For example, only one site (Utica) has staged an event which directly confronted the tobacco interests. No sites have made use of the counter-arguing strategies in debates because there have been limited if any opportunities in the media.

The reasons for this limited use of media advocacy are generally two-fold. First, there is often a limited base of experience to draw on in working with the media. There is some reticence to get on the phone with or visit local broadcast and print newspeople. The general approach to making use of local media outlets is a passive one. Second, and more fundamentally, there appears to be an unwillingness on the part of community members and organizations to be cast in a confrontational role.

This latter attitude is not unexpected. Most communities make decisions through a process of consensus, not confrontation. The overall philosophy of COMMIT is based on consensus building and coalition development as a primary change strategy. The media advocacy technique tends to fit more with a strategy that assumes conflict between competing interests and seeks to stimulate people to take action on a policy level. For example, few communities would not support the use of media to inform smokers about the danger of cigarette smoking and resources for quitting. On the other hand, the use of media to promote policy change or challenge the ethics and legitimacy of the tobacco industry can often create anxiety. The proactive, sometimes aggressive quality of media advocacy has resulted in limited, strategic use by COMMIT communities.

The two brief case studies presented here illustrate various pieces of media advocacy. For example, the use of creative epidemiology can be seen in the way that Utica took existing mortality data and linked it to market share of the tobacco company. In the Oregon site several activities built on existing national news stories and localized and personalized these stories with local angles. In general, both sites directed activities toward reframing tobacco issues from one of simply an individual problem to one of community wide interest with a focus on social policy.

The comprehensive evaluation integral to COMMIT insures that a great deal will be learned about media advocacy and the general use of mass media by community groups. One key lesson that has already emerged is that media strategies, like other approaches, must be consistent with the values of the community. Media advocacy provides a number of useful tactics and offers an overall strategy to guide the use of mass media. However, for many communities the confrontational and proactive posture of media advocacy may limit its attractiveness.

Finally, COMMIT represents the first wide-scale effort to train media advocates at the local level. The experience to date suggests the preliminary conclusion that the skills needed by the media advocate may be too complex to communicate in a simple training. The policy advocacy perspective may require ongoing technical assistance and stronger support systems in the advocates' community.

REFERENCES

1. U.S. Surgeon General, *Reducing the Health Consequences of Smoking: 25 Years of Progress*, Public Health Service, Centers for Disease Control, Center for Chronic Disease Prevention and Health Promotion, Office on Smoking and Health, DHHS Publication No. (CDC) 89-8411, 1989.
2. P. Hilts, Smokers' Health Toll Put at $52 Billion, *New York Times* (National), p. A 12, February 21, 1990.
3. D. Yach, The Impact of Smoking in Developing Countries with Special Reference to Africa, *International Journal of Health Services, 16*:2, pp. 279-292, 1986.
4. R. Masironi, Smoking Trends Worldwide, in *Abstracts*, Seventh World Conference on Tobacco and Health, Perth, Australia, p. 67, April 1990.
5. R. Peto, The Future Worldwide Health Effects of Current Smoking Patterns: WHO Consultative Group Estimates for the 1990s and Beyond, paper presented at the Seventh World Conference on Smoking and Health, Perth, Australia, April 1990.
6. M. Mattson, et al., Evaluation Plan for the Community Intervention Trial for Smoking Cessation (COMMIT), *International Quarterly of Community Health Education, 11*:3, pp. 271-290, 1990-91.
7. K. Corbett, et al., Process Evaluation in the Community Intervention Trial for Smoking Cessation (COMMIT), *International Quarterly of Community Health Education, 11*:3, pp. 291-309, 1990-91.

8. B. Thompson, et al., Principles of Community Organization and Partnership for Smoking Cessation in the Community Intervention Trial for Smoking Cessation (COMMIT), *International Quarterly of Community Health Education, 11*:3, pp. 187-203, 1990-91.

9. J. Ockene, et al., Health Care Providers as Key Change Agents in the Community Intervention Trial for Smoking Cessation (COMMIT), *International Quarterly of Community Health Education, 11*:3, pp. 223-237, 1990-91.

10. P. Pomrehn, et al., Enhancing Resources for Smoking Cessation through Community Intervention: COMMIT as a Prototype, *International Quarterly of Community Health Education, 11*:3, pp. 259-269, 1990-91.

11. G. Sorensen, et al., Promoting Smoking Control through Worksites in the Community Intervention Trial for Smoking Cessation (COMMIT), *International Quarterly of Community Health Education, 11*:3, pp. 239-257, 1990-91.

12. K. Warner, *Selling Smoke: Cigarette Advertising and Public Health*, American Public Health Association, Washington, D.C., 1986.

13. B. Seldon and K. Doroodian, A Simultaneous Model of Cigarette Advertising: Effects on Demand and Industry Response to Public Policy, *The Review of Economics and Statistics, LXXI*, pp. 673-677, November 1989.

14. J. Tye, K. Warner, and S. Glantz, Tobacco Advertising and Consumption: Evidence of a Causal Relationship, *Journal of Public Health Policy, 8*:4, pp. 492-508, 1987.

15. W. Weis and C. Burke, Media Content and Tobacco Advertising: An Unhealthy Addiction, *Journal of Communication, 36*:4, pp. 59-69, 1986.

16. M. Minkler, L. Wallack, and P. Madden, Alcohol and Cigarette Advertising in *Ms.* Magazine, *Journal of Public Health Policy, 8*:2, pp. 164-179, 1987.

17. L. Kessler, Women's Magazines' Coverage of Smoking Related Hazards, *Journalism Quarterly, 66*:2, pp. 316-323, 1989.

18. K. Warner, The Effects of the Anti-Smoking Campaign on Cigarette Consumption, *American Journal of Public Health, 67*:7, pp. 645-650, 1977.

19. B. Flay, *Selling the Smokeless Society: Fifty-Six Evaluated Mass Media Programs and Campaigns Worldwide*, American Public Health Association, Washington, D.C., 1987.

20. B. Flay, Mass Media and Smoking Cessation: A Critical Review, *American Journal of Public Health, 77*:2, pp. 153-160, 1987.

21. K. Cummings, R. Sciandra, and S. Markello, Impact of a Newspaper-Mediated Quit Smoking Program, *American Journal of Public Health, 77*, pp. 1452-1453, 1987.

22. J. Pierce, P. Macaskill, and D. Hill, Long-Term Effectiveness on Mass Media Led Antismoking Campaigns in Australia, *American Journal of Public Health, 80*:5, pp. 565-569, 1990.

23. K. Cummings, R. Sciandra, S. Davis, and B. Rimer, Response to an Anti-Smoking Campaign Aimed at Mothers with Young Children, *Health Education Research, 4*, pp. 429-437, 1989.

24. A. Freedman, New Smoke from RJR Under Fire, *Wall Street Journal*, p. B1, February 20, 1990.

25. M. Specter and P. Farhi, Critics Say Results of Targeted Tobacco Sales Pitches Are Deadly, *Washington Post*, p. A4, January 21, 1990.

26. An Uproar Over Billboards in Poor Areas, *New York Times*, p. D10, May 1, 1989.

27. Fighting Ads in the Inner City, *Newsweek*, p. 46, February 5, 1990.
28. S. Strom, Switching Ads Rather than Fighting, *New York Times* (National), p. A8, April 10, 1990.
29. *Media Strategies for Smoking Control Guidelines*, U.S. Department of Health and Human Services, Public Health Service, National Institutes of Health, Publication No. 89-3013, March 1989.
30. *Smoke Signals: The Smoking Control Handbook*, prepared for the American Cancer Society by the Advocacy Institute, 1987.
31. L. Brown, Hype in a Good Cause, *Channels*, 7:7, p. 26, 1987.

Direct reprint requests to:

Lawrence Wallack
516 Warren Hall
School of Public Health
University of California
Berkeley, CA 94720

HEALTH CARE PROVIDERS AS KEY CHANGE AGENTS IN THE COMMUNITY INTERVENTION TRIAL FOR SMOKING CESSATION (COMMIT)

JUDITH K. OCKENE, PH.D.
University of Massachusetts Medical School, Worcester

ELIZABETH LINDSAY, PH.D.
McMaster University
Hamilton, Ontario

LAWRENCE BERGER, M.D., M.P.H.
Lovelace Medical Foundation
Albuquerque, New Mexico

NORMAN HYMOWITZ, PH.D.
University of Medicine and Dentistry of New Jersey, Newark

For the COMMIT Research Group

ABSTRACT

The Community Intervention Trial for Smoking Cessation (COMMIT) is a multi-center collaborative trial sponsored by the National Cancer Institute. COMMIT utilizes multiple, community-based channels to facilitate quit attempts among heavy cigarette smokers. The "health care provider channel" is important, in that physicians, dentists, and other health care providers can effect changes in smoking behavior at both the individual and community level. There are over 1,600 primary care physicians and general practice dentists in the COMMIT intervention communities. This article describes the conceptual basis for the health care provider activities; results of a survey of

Int'l. Quarterly of Community Health Education, Vol. 11(3) 223-237, 1990-91

© 1991, Baywood Publishing Co., Inc.

community attitudes and behaviors regarding smoking and health care; specific training and intervention activities; and the role of health care providers as community change agents in the smoking cessation arena.

COMMIT BACKGROUND

The Community Intervention Trial for Smoking Cessation (COMMIT) is a multi-center collaborative randomized trial, which tests the effect of coordinated community-wide smoking cessation activities on cessation rates. It is funded by the National Cancer Institute and involves eleven matched pairs of intervention and control communities in the United States and Canada. Descriptions of the design and evaluation plan and the community mobilization process required for community support are presented elsewhere [1, 2].

The COMMIT protocol describes specific activities which occur in all eleven intervention communities and are delivered through several channels or sectors within the communities. To ensure community participation, a Community Board and four Task Forces plan and implement the COMMIT intervention protocol with the assistance of COMMIT staff. The Health Care Provider Task Force, made up of leaders from the health care community, tailors the intervention activities for their specific community.

In this article we summarize the methods and reasoning used in COMMIT for planning interventions aimed at health care providers; the goals for health care providers; and describe the intervention protocol and activities during the first two years of implementation. In addition, we provide data describing perceptions of community residents regarding the role of physicians and dentists in smoking intervention.

THE ROLE OF HEALTH CARE PROVIDERS

Physicians and other health care professionals, as credible sources of smoking and health information, can take advantage of clinical opportunities to motivate patients and influence change in smoking, both at the individual patient level and at a broader community level. Since 70 percent of smokers see their physician at least once per year [3] and 62 percent of patients see their dentists at least once per year [4], physicians and dentists have the opportunity to reach a large number of smokers. To capitalize on this opportunity COMMIT promotes smoking interventions which physicians and dental care professionals can integrate into their usual office practice routine.

Physicians and other health professionals have a history of involvement in the smoking and health arena [5-10]. In addition, recent advances in pharmacologic therapy and behavioral counseling provide new opportunities for them to have an impact. Several recently completed, randomized controlled trials have demonstrated that physicians and dentists can have an impact on smokers' cessation rates. These studies provided guidance for the selection of COMMIT activities for physicians and dentists [11-18].

Three of the trials [15, 17, 18] collectively demonstrated that physicians who receive special training to assist smokers during the course of regular medical encounters have a greater effect on the smoking behavior of their patients than physicians not so trained [19-21]. Studies have also demonstrated that physicians who are prompted or cued to intervene, such as with a reminder affixed to the front of the chart, have a greater effect on the smoking behavior of their patients than do physicians not so cued [11, 15, 17, 18].

The studies provide support for the conclusion that when physicians are taught to use specific smoking intervention skills, cessation rates increase significantly; cueing alone does not have as strong an effect as cueing combined with training in the use of smoking intervention skills. Those physician-delivered smoking intervention studies that included both training of physicians and staff, and implementation of an office system which cued the physician to intervene and provide followup, produced the best cessation results [17, 18]. In an effort to apply the best available interventions, COMMIT activities focus on training physicians and dental care teams to apply effective clinical strategies, and on the implementation of office systems which cue and support smoking intervention.

Few studies have assessed the effectiveness of interventions delivered by dental care teams [11, 22]. However, the work that has been done in smoking cessation [12], as well as preventive dentistry in general [22], provided a rationale for the inclusion of the dental focus within the health care provider channel. Other health care professionals, nurses and chiropractors for example, are being invited to participate in the project, but the lack of intervention research with these professional groups led to their exclusion from the mandated elements of the protocol.

Another major effort of the COMMIT health care provider channel is devoted to the adoption and implementation of smoke-free policies by hospitals, medical offices, and other health care facilities. Smoke-free health care facilities can be successfully promoted, and they provide a healthy model to the community for smoke-free worksites and have the potential to reach many smokers [23-27]. There is a strong movement towards smoke-free health care nationwide. Similar kinds of policy initiatives in COMMIT intervention communities contribute to the success of the community effort.

The COMMIT baseline survey [1] of randomly selected residents in the eleven matched pairs of communities demonstrated that approximately three quarters of smokers have visited their physician and over 60 percent had seen their dentist in the past year. A high proportion believed that it is likely or very likely that they will suffer a serious health problem if they continue to smoke and approximately 60 percent believed that smoking already was affecting their health adversely. Over three quarters believed that stopping smoking will likely decrease their chances of having serious health problems in the future and that if their doctor told them to stop smoking they would try (Table 1). However, only 39 percent reported

Table 1. The Frequency of Visits of Physicians and Dentists, Perceptions of Health Status and the Role of Physicians and Dentists in Smoking Cessation as Assessed by a Community Cross-Sectional Survey

	Heavy Smokers[a] (%)	Light/Moderate Smokers[b] (%)
Have visited physician in past 12 months	73[c]	76
Have visited dentist in past 12 months	64	68
Likely or very likely to have serious health problem from smoking, if continue	83	77
Likely or very likely to decrease risk of serious health problem if stop smoking	82	85
Smoking has already affected health	60	62
If doctor told you to stop you would try	71	81
If dentist told you to stop you would try	45	56
You have asked your doctor or dentist to help you stop smoking	18	13

Source: COMMIT Evaluation Survey, 1989.
[a] Smoke ≥ 25 cigarettes/day.
[b] Smoke < 25 cigarettes/day.
[c] Numbers have been rounded to nearest percent.

being told by their physician and/or dentist to stop smoking; 11 percent of these were by dentists, 78 percent by physicians and 10 percent by both (Table 2). In addition, only approximately 15 percent have asked their physician or dentist for help to stop smoking (Table 1). Thus, the smokers in the COMMIT communities believe that health care providers can have an impact on their smoking behavior but generally patients have not sought nor providers offered such help.

Table 2 displays other practices of physicians and dentists reported by community residents in the baseline survey. In general, dentists were less active than were physicians. For example, approximately 67 percent of smokers noted that in the past year they were asked by their physician or dentist whether they were smokers: approximately 15 percent of these were asked by their dentists. Since previously noted research has demonstrated that health care provider interventions can be effective in helping smokers to quit, there is much room for increased implementation of smoking intervention practices by physicians and dentists.

Table 2. Smokers Reported Frequency in Past Twelve Months of Specific
Elements of Smoking Cessation Intervention by Physicians and Dentists
in the Intervention Communities (All Smokers)

| | | If Yes, Who? | | |
	Yes (%)	Physicians (%)	Dentists (%)	Both (%)
Asked me if I smoked	67	58	15	27
Explained the dangers of smoking	49	72	13	15
Told me to stop smoking	39	78	11	11
Suggested I set a specific date to stop smoking	9	82	6	12
Gave me a pamphlet about smoking	19	85	17	8
Prescribed nicotine gum	12	92	8	0
Referred me to a stop-smoking program	5	90	8	2
Asked me to return for a visit to discuss smoking	4	94	4	2

Source: COMMIT Evaluation Survey, 1989.
[a] Numbers have been rounded to nearest percent.

GOALS FOR HEALTH CARE PROVIDERS

Based on the understanding of how health care providers can influence smoking cessation the following overall goals were set to guide activities in this channel:

1. Health care providers will be aware of, promote, and play an active role in smoking intervention efforts in the community;
2. Health care providers will regard smoking cessation advice as the minimal standard of practice; some providers will go beyond providing advice;
3. All health care facilities will adopt and effectively implement policies for a smoke-free environment; and
4. Smoking patients will more actively seek assistance from the health care system to stop smoking.

Table 3. Health Care Provider Task Force

Impact Objectives

---

1. Among heavy smokers who have visited a physician or dentist in the past twelve months increase the percentage who report having been told to stop smoking or asked to set a quit date by their physician or dentist.

    *   1993 60 percent of smokers will report having been told by a physician and 35 percent by a dentist to stop smoking

    *   1993 25 percent of smokers will report having been asked to set a date for stopping smoking by a physician and 20 percent by a dentist

2. Increase the percentage of physicians and dentists who report setting stop smoking dates with patients most of the time

    *   1993 25 percent of physicans and 20 percent of dentists will report setting stop smoking dates with patients most of the time

3. Increase the percentage of health care facilities (e.g., doctors/dentist offices, clinics, hospitals) that do not allow smoking by either patients or staff

    *   1993 90 percent of physicians and dentists offices and other health care facilities will be smoke-free

---

INTERVENTION PROTOCOL

To achieve these specific goals activities were developed and impact objectives and timelines established. Table 3 presents the impact objectives. COMMIT evaluation surveys [1] measure progress in achieving such impact objectives but these data are not yet available. Primary care physicians and dentists are the focus of the health care provider protocol because they see the largest percentage of smokers, and they are generally receptive to doing preventive interventions. Targeted physician groups include the primary care specialties of internal/general medicine, family practice, obstetrics/gynecology and osteopathy. Targeted dental offices are those practicing general dentistry.

The protocol requires activities which: educate practicing physicians and dental health teams; involve them in promoting community-wide smoking control activities; and establish smoke-free offices and hospitals. Table 4 presents the required activities for this channel. Whenever possible, linkages between other channel activities in the protocol are promoted in order to reinforce the effects. For example, both the Smokers' Network and local cessation program guides, both of

Table 4. Health Care Provider Task Force

Intervention Activities
Training leaders for basic and comprehensive continuing education sessions for physicians and dental health professionals
Providing basic continuing education sessions for physicians
Providing comprehensive continuing education sessions for physicians
Providing basic continuing education sessions for dental health professionals
Providing comprehensive continuing education sessions for dental health professionals
Strategies for motivating and training office staff
Promotion of smokers' network
Influential training of physicians and dental health professionals
Promotion of smoke-free policies in health care facilities

which are primarily Cessation Resources Activities [28], are actively promoted through health care settings.

Some communities are finding that other health professionals such as pharmacists, and occupational and public health nurses are ready and able to reach smokers and have chosen to include them in COMMIT activities. For example, in the Canadian site, chiropractors attended training events with family physicians, and physician leaders provided special events for public health nurses.

Approximately thirty physician and thirty dental offices were randomly selected in each community and office staff in these practices were surveyed by telephone in 1990 and asked about office smoking policies and available cessation resources (Impact Objectives 2 and 3 in Table 3). Mailed surveys were sent to all primary care physicians and general practice dentists to determine their counseling cessation practices. More information on these surveys is presented elsewhere [1].

Physician and Dental Training

There are three levels of training activities provided for physicians and dental care teams designed to achieve the educational goals and facilitate regular counseling of all smokers following a standard protocol.

The *most advanced level of training* develops leadership and educational skills for medical and dental care teams within the intervention communities. This *"train the trainers"* approach uses national training activities to build the capacity of medical and dental care teams within the communities to deliver the other two levels of training.

One or two physicians from each of the intervention communities attended a National training session in January 1989 and learned how to deliver both the one hour introductory type of session as well as the longer skill development workshop. These physicians have served as training resources in providing CME opportunities for physicians during the 1990 program year. Parallel training was also provided for a dentist and dental hygienist from each community.

National experts in the clinical aspects of smoking cessation designed the materials for the train-the-trainers workshops and serve as the instructors [29-31]. The workshop provided both information and experience in conducting comprehensive training workshops in the local communities. Particular emphasis was placed on how to provide supportive feedback and how to facilitate practice of intervention strategies through role playing, simulated patients, and other experiential techniques. These advanced workshops continue to be offered by NCI in conjunction with regional and national professional meetings, to encourage participation by community health providers.

Basic training is a 40-60 minute presentation by local health care providers who attended the National training and by invited guest speakers. It is intended to motivate physicians and dentists to intervene with smokers and to promote interest in more comprehensive, advanced training.

The following areas are emphasized:

- the health benefits of smoking cessation;
- importance and effectiveness of health care provider intervention;
- how to create an office environment and practice that supports smoking cessation and maintenance;
- a brief summary of intervention strategies;
- factors which often interfere with maintaining cessation and how to address them; and
- steps to further develop clinical skills in cessation counseling.

The presentations are incorporated into existing networks for professional development and continuing education, such as grand rounds at local hospitals and regular meeting of professional organizations.

Comprehensive training offers more detailed instruction and demonstrations for how to create and deliver effective smoking cessation interventions in physicians and dentists' offices. This training includes modeling and role-playing to practice smoking intervention skills and build on the content of the basic training. Attendees receive a manual instructing them in the physician-delivered smoking intervention steps [30].

In order to help physicians/dental care teams develop smoking cessation plans with patients, they are taught to use those elements found to be most appropriate and effective within a health care setting. Health care providers are trained to: ASK questions to find out if someone smokes and whether he/she is interested in trying to stop; ADVISE patients to stop smoking by providing personally relevant, health related reasons for cessation; ASSIST individuals to stop smoking by helping them to set a stop smoking date, recommending that patients make a plan to stop, as well as provide other specific aids such as the offer of a prescription of nicotine gum if deemed appropriate and the provisions of self-help materials; and ARRANGE for further follow-up support through telephone calls or return visits for appropriate patients.

The training for the dental care team follows a format similar to the physician training but with a greater emphasis on the role of the dental assistant or hygienist. Both dentists and an assistant or hygienist have attended training in intervention procedures and planning office routines. They were provided with an instructional manual [32] and other resource materials are also available (e.g., [33]).

There are a total of 909 primary care physicians ($\bar{x}$ = 83/community) and 731 general practice dentists ($\bar{x}$ = 66/community) in the intervention communities. During the four years of intervention, a major goal is to attract 80 percent (727) of primary care physicians and 65 percent (475) of general care dentists to training events. All sites have conducted health care provider training and at this stage of the study, 45 percent (approximately 400) of primary care physicians and 15 percent (100) of dentists have received basic training.

Influential Activities

Each community, through a community analysis, has identified influential health care professionals who are interested in smoking as a community health problem. In addition to their involvement in continuing medical and dental education, influentials' opportunities for community change include promoting smoke-free health care facilities; supporting new regulations–and the enforcement of existing regulations–about sale of tobacco to minors, and smoking in public places, schools, and worksites; and serving as spokespersons with the media, schools and community groups. COMMIT staff provide assistance to health care provider "influentials" in the form of a training manual with learning resources [34]; materials from DOC [35] a national physical group involved in innovative– and often humorous–anti-tobacco activities [35]; and materials and training in media and legislative advocacy [36-39].

Smoke-Free Health Care Facilities

The intervention protocol requires the promotion of smoke-free policies in all health care facilities including hospitals, clinics, and medical and dental offices. COMMIT staff and volunteers facilitate policy development and provide resources to encourage smoke-free environments. The first step in this process was to build the commitment of physicians and dentists to initiate and support these policies. While this occurs to some extent as part of the training events provided in the community, it has been slow to develop in several sites.

Both establishing policies and enforcing them requires careful planning and a "team approach." From the outset, it was important to involve representatives of all the groups that will be affected by policy changes [36, 40]. Smoke-free policies at hospitals and other large health-care facilities sometimes raise sensitive labor-management issues or fears that a facility's "market competitiveness" will be impaired. Office staff may themselves be smokers and need to have their concerns expressed and supportively addressed.

Smokers are generally less supportive than non-smokers of non-smoking policies in hospitals and doctors' offices and heavy smokers in particular express the need for designated smoking areas. However, a policy which does not allow smoking in doctors' offices was supported by approximately 63 percent of heavy smokers as assessed in the baseline survey [1] of community residents.

TAILORING THE INTERVENTION TO THE COMMUNITY

The above intervention activities are incorporated into the community-wide interventions implemented by COMMIT. The health care providers' intervention protocol is tailored to each community by the Health Care Providers Task Force through the development of the Annual Action Plans. The Task Force develops a plan each year to determine: which activities need to be implemented; how this will occur; who will do it; and what resources are needed; and a timeline for completion of tasks. This local development of the plan encourages community ownership of protocol activities.

After randomization, an in-depth analysis occurred in the intervention communities [2]. Interviews with influential health care providers, including individuals involved in continuing education for providers, provided information which helped tailor the intervention to communities. The community's health care priorities and history of concerns were also investigated. The community analysis assisted in the formation of the Community Board and Health Care Task Force in the intervention communities by identifying leaders from the health care sector.

There can be wide variation in the nature and needs of health care providers in different communities. The scheduling of COMMIT events, such as training workshops, is arranged to accommodate the hectic work schedules experienced by most health care providers. They are held in the early morning, evening or on the weekend. Basic training is usually embedded in naturally occurring "grand rounds" or medical meetings. A range of incentives–continuing education credits, spouse events, gourmet meals–have proved necessary to attract participants to the longer comprehensive training.

Implementing the health care provider activities at some sites has been difficult. Physicians and dentists who take an active role in smoking cessation are not always in the mainstream of their professional communities. In all communities it has been challenging to attract busy health care providers to half day training events in their own community. They may prefer instead to obtain their educational credits at a major conference out-of-town. Corbett et al. present more detail on how sites have fared in recruiting providers for comprehensive training [41]. Literature on smoking cessation competes with an enormous volume of reading material–both scholarly and promotional–that regularly inundates medical and dental offices. Barriers to interventions are continually being dealt with in the communities. For example, in Fitchburg/Leominister, Massachusetts, a pulmonary physician wrote to each of his medical colleagues at his hospital suggesting that they lunch together and discuss the barriers to smoking intervention in their practices, methods to deal with these barriers, and how to intervene with smokers. He has had several colleagues who responded well to the idea and met with him. This physician had originally been skeptical of the effectiveness of intervention until he tried it. Another physician on the board, a DOC member who had been very interested in minors' access to tobacco, has produced his own videotape concerning this problem and has presented this to his colleagues and encouraged their interest in smoking intervention.

In Santa Fe, New Mexico, the task force produced a videotape entitled, "You can make a difference," which was used for basic training. Starring roles were performed by the health department physician, chairman of the DOC chapter, hospital administrator, president of the medical society, and a prominent local cardiologist. The use of local personalities, humor and community setting were intended to maintain viewer interest.

Several communities have initiated newsletters for health care providers. For example, the inaugural issue of the Santa Fe newsletter, "Smoke-Free Signals," discussed diagnostic codes to consider for reimbursement of smoking cessation counseling. To address the reimbursement issue at the Canadian site, the Task Force appealed successfully to the provincial government to ensure that physician-delivered smoking interventions will be reimbursed by the Province's health insurance plan.

In most communities there has been a strong interest from health care professionals other than physicians and dentists. In Paterson, New Jersey, health workers in the hypertension screening program have access to many smokers who otherwise might not be reached by office-based programs. Therefore, COMMIT staff work along with the hypertension screening program, arranging to deliver messages and materials on smoking as well as high blood pressure. Several sites have many "alternative providers" such as chiropractors, acupuncturists, naturopaths, and herbalists. Individual COMMIT sites sponsor special training workshops, organize task force subcommittees to include a range of providers, and prepare unique professional education materials. For example, in the Canadian site, chiropractors attended training events with family physicians and physician leaders provided special events for public health nurses. At the Medford/Ashland, Oregon site, a chiropractor is a task force member and has presented at comprehensive physician trainings. At several sites such as Bellingham, special events have been held for the nursing community.

Patient populations in different communities may have unique requirements and smoking cessation materials have been designed for non-English speakers in several communities. In Santa Fe, older-age smokers have been targeted through a collaboration by the COMMIT project and the State's Agency on Aging: a smoking cessation self-help manual was created for elderly persons who are visited in their homes by health care workers. A "prenatal smoking cessation initiative" is being designed by representatives of the WIC (Women/Infant/Children) nutrition bureau, a neighborhood clinic for low-income people, COMMIT project staff and pediatricians, and the state Lung Association.

DISCUSSION AND CONCLUSIONS

Physicians, dentists, and other health care providers can serve as role models, advocate for more healthy environments, and encourage smokers to quit. Given that a large percentage of heavy smokers visit a physician and/or dentist each year, the clinician's role in facilitating smoking cessation is important from both a clinical and public health perspective. The results of the COMMIT baseline evaluation survey confirms the importance of health care providers in the smoking cessation effort. Most smokers are aware that smoking is harmful to their health, and state that they would try to stop smoking if told to do so by their physicians. The general public is very supportive of non-smoking norms for health care facilities, and many smokers, too, agree that smoking should at least be restricted in such settings.

Given these considerations, there is considerable logic to the COMMIT protocol for the health care channel. Key goals are to train physicians, dentists, and other health care professionals to counsel or advise smokers to stop smoking, to set up their office practice to facilitate smoking intervention, and advocate for smoke-free health care facilities and other smoking-related legislation.

Health care providers affect their colleagues' response and professional norms through their leadership roles as members of the COMMIT Community Board, Health Care Task Force, and as representatives of their own professional societies and agencies. Not all health care providers are participating and barriers exist to the integration into practice of systematic, effective smoking interventions. These barriers include time constraints; provider skepticism that they can "really make a difference" in getting smokers to quit; competing demands; and limited training in cessation counseling techniques [3]. However, the educational events and materials provided to health care professionals not only build skills in working with smokers but also demonstrate how to integrate this work into regular office routines.

The COMMIT intervention is built on the premise that the interaction of many activities will magnify the impact of any one approach. The mobilizing of the health care community and their active participation throughout the program will increase the chances of achieving trial goals and of having a significant impact on smoking cessation.

REFERENCES

1. M. E. Mattson, K. M. Cummings, W. R. Lynn, C. Giffen, D. Corle, and T. Pechacek, Evaluation Plan for the Community Intervention Trial for Smoking Cessation (COMMIT), *International Quarterly of Community Health Education, 11*:3, pp. 271-290, 1990-91.
2. B. Thompson, L. Wallack, E. Lichtenstein, and T. Pechacek, Principles of Community Organization and Partnership for Smoking Cessation in the Community Intervention Trial for Smoking Cessation (COMMIT), *International Quarterly of Community Health Education, 11*:3, pp. 187-203, 1990-91.
3. J. K. Ockene, Physician Delivered Interventions for Smoking Cessation: Strategies for Increasing Effectiveness, *Preventive Medicine, 7*, pp. 723-737, 1987.
4. U.S. Department of Health and Human Services, *Reducing the Health Consequences of Smoking: 25 Years of Progress. A Report of the Surgeon General*, U.S. Department of Health and Human Services, Public Health Service, Centers for Disease Control, Center for Chronic Disease Prevention and Health Promotion, Office on Smoking and Health, DHHS Publication No. (CDC) 89-8411, 1989.
5. D. T. Frederickson, How to Help Your Patients Stop Smoking–Guidelines for the Office Physician, *Diseases of the Chest, 54*, pp. 28-34, 1968.
6. N. Hymowitz, The Practicing Physician and Smoking Cessation, *The Journal of the Medical Society of New Jersey, 74*, pp. 139-141, 1977.
7. J. K. Ockene, Nine Ways to Help Your Patients Stop Smoking, *Your Patient and Cancer*, 1982.
8. Royal College of Physicians of London, *Smoking and Health*, Pitman, London, 1971.
9. M. A. H. Russell, Cigarette Dependence: II-Doctor's Role in Management, *British Medical Journal, 2*, pp. 393-395, 1971.
10. J. L. Steinfeld, The Physician's Role: The Physician's Responsibility to His Smoking Patient, *Rhode Island Medical Journal, 55*, pp. 119-123, 1972.
11. S. J. Cohen, A. G. Christen, B. P. Katz, et al., Counseling Medical and Dental Patients about Cigarette Smoking: The Impact of Nicotine Gum and Chart Reminders, *American Journal of Public Health, 77*, pp. 313-316, 1987.
12. S. J. Cohen, G. K. Stookey, B. P. Katz, et al., Helping Smokers Quit: A Randomized Controlled Trial with Private Practice Dentists, *Journal of the American Dental Association, 118*, pp. 41-45, 1989.

13. S. Cohen, G. Stookey, B. Katz, et al., Encouraging Primary Care Physicians to Help Smokers Quit, *Annals of Internal Medicine, 110*, pp. 648-652, 1989.
14. S. Cummings, T. Coates, R. Richard, et al., Training Physicians in Counseling about Smoking Cessation: A Randomized Trial of the "Quit for Life" Program, *Annals of Internal Medicine, 110*, pp. 640-647, 1989.
15. N. K. Janz, M. H. Becker, J. P. Kirsch, S. A. Eraker, J. E. Billi, and J. O. Woolliscroft, Evaluation of a Minimal-Contact Smoking Cessation Intervention in an Outpatient Setting, *American Journal of Public Health, 77*, pp. 849-851, 1987.
16. T. E Kottke, M. L. Brekke, L. I. Solberg, and J. R. Hughes, A Randomized Trial to Increase Smoking Intervention by Physicians, *Journal of the American Medical Association, 261*:14, pp. 2101-2106, 1989.
17. J. K. Ockene, J. Kristeller, R. Goldberg, et al., Increasing the Efficacy of Physician-Delivered Smoking Intervention: A Randomized Clinical Trial, *Journal of General Internal Medicine*, in press.
18. D. Wilson, W. Taylor, R. Gilbert, et al., A Randomized Trial of a Family Physician Intervention for Smoking Cessation, *Journal of the American Medical Association, 260*, pp. 1570-1574, 1988.
19. J. R. Gilbert, D. M. Wilson, J. S. Singer, et al., A Family Physician Smoking Cessation Program: An Evaluation of the Role of Follow-Up Visits, (manuscript submitted).
20. E. A. Lindsay, D. M. Wilson, A. J. Best, et al., A Randomized Trial of Physicians Training for Smoking Cessation, *American Journal of Health Practices, 3*:3, pp. 11-18, 1988.
21. J. K. Ockene, M. E. Quirk, R. J. Goldberg, et al., A Residents' Training Program for the Development of Smoking Intervention Skills, *Archives of Internal Medicine, 148*, pp. 1039-1045, 1988.
22. B. Gerber, T. Coates, L. Zahnd, et al., Dentists as Smoking Cessation Counsellors, *Journal of the American Dental Association, 118*, pp. 29-32, 1989.
23. J. L. Andrews, Reducing Smoking in the Hospital. An Effective Model Program, *CHEST, 84*, pp. 206-209, 1983.
24. H. H. Dawley, The Discouragement of Smoking in a Hospital Setting: The Importance of Modeled Behavior, *The International Journal of the Addictions, 16*, pp. 905-910, 1981.
25. J. M. Knapp and T. E. Kottke, The Achievement of Clean Air Health Care: Is It Appropriate? Is It Feasible?, *Archives of Internal Medicine*, in press.
26. T. E. Kottke, *Clean Air Health Care–A Guide to Establishing Smoke-Free Health Care Facilities*, Department of Medicine, University of Minnesota, 1986.
27. G. Sorensen and J. K. Ockene, Non-Smoking Policies for Hospitals, *Archives of Internal Medicine*, in press.
28. P. Pomrehn, R. Sciandra, R. Shipley, W. Lynn, and H. Lando, Enhancing Resources for Smoking Cessation through Community Intervention: COMMIT As a Prototype, *International Quarterly of Community Health Education, 11*:3, pp. 259-269, 1990-91.
29. U.S. Department of Health and Human Services, *How to Help Your Patients Stop Smoking: Trainer's Guide*, Public Health Service, National Institutes of Health, 1990.
30. T. J. Glynn and N. W. Manley, *How to Help Your Patients Stop Smoking: A National Cancer Institute Manual for Physicians*, U.S. Department of Health and Human Services, Public Health Service, National Institutes of Health, 1989.

31. J. K. Ockene, J. Kristeller, and K. Kalan, *Physician-Delivered Smoking Intervention Program: Facilitator's Guide*, University of Massachusetts Medical School, Worcester, MA, 1988.
32. U.S. Department of Health and Human Services, *How to Help Your Patients Stop Using Tobacco: Dental Trainer's Guide*, National Institutes of Health Services, 1990.
33. H. S. Borden, A. G. Christen, J. L. McDonald, et al., A Smoking Cessation Program for the Oral Health Care Practice, *Dental Hygiene, 62*, pp. 339-343, 1988.
34. L. R. Berger, Manual for Training Health Care "Influentials," Prepared for the COMMIT Project, National Cancer Institute, January 1989.
35. Doctors Ought to Care, Special edition on Medical Activism, *DOC News and Views*, Summer 1989.
36. American Medical Association, *Creating a Tobacco-Free Society: A Physician Leadership Kit*, Chicago, 1987.
37. Medicinema Limited, *Lobbying for Lives: Lessons from the Front*, 30-minute color video, 131 Albany Avenue, Toronto, Canada M5R-3C5.
38. National Cancer Institute, *Media Strategies for Smoking Control: Guidelines from a Consensus Workshop*, NIH Publication No. 89-3013, March 1989.
39. M. Pertschuk, The Physician as Health Promotion Media Advocate, Presentation to the Robert Wood Johnson Foundation Clinical Scholars Program, Available from the Advocacy Institute, 1730 Rhode Island Avenue, N.W., Suite 600, Washington, D.C. 20036-3118, October 1988.
40. T. E. Kottke, C. Hill, C. Heitzig, et al., Smoke-Free Hospitals, *Minnesota Medicine, 68*, pp. 53-55, 1985.
41. K. Corbett, B. Thompson, N. White, and M. Taylor, Process Evaluation in the Community Intervention Trial for Smoking Cessation (COMMIT), *International Quarterly of Community Health Education, 11*:3, pp. 291-309, 1990-91.

Direct reprint requests to:

Judith K. Ockene, Ph.D.
University of Massachusetts Medical School
Department of Medicine
Preventive and Behavioral Medicine
55 Lake Avenue, North
Worcester, MA 01655

PROMOTING SMOKING CONTROL THROUGH WORKSITES IN THE COMMUNITY INTERVENTION TRIAL FOR SMOKING CESSATION (COMMIT)

GLORIAN SORENSEN, PH.D., M.P.H.
University of Massachusetts Medical School, Worcester

RUSSELL E. GLASGOW, PH.D.
Oregon Research Institute, Eugene

KITTY CORBETT, PH.D., M.P.H.
Kaiser Permanente Medical Care Program
Oakland, California

For the COMMIT Research Group

ABSTRACT

This article describes the worksite intervention and assessment aspects of the COMMIT project. Following a brief review of the rationale for worksite smoking control efforts and how planning for such activities can be conducted as part of community-based interventions, we describe the COMMIT worksite protocol. All intervention communities conduct specified activities in the areas of smoking policy, motivational and incentive procedures to encourage smoking cessation, and provision of self-help materials and cessation services for employees. Assessment procedures include a computerized process objectives system, surveys of worksites in each of the 22 COMMIT communities, and work related questions on surveys of community residents. Baseline data that have informed the process objectives for the worksite channel are presented, as are examples of how intervention activities have been tailored to different communities.

Although cigarette smoking is on the decline overall within the United States, cessation rates remain low among heavy smokers and among less educated groups

Int'l. Quarterly of Community Health Education, Vol. 11(3) 239-257, 1990-91

© 1991, Baywood Publishing Co., Inc.

[1, 2]. Changes in social norms and community-wide support for nonsmoking may be an effective strategy for promoting cessation among these groups. The Community Intervention Trial for Smoking Cessation (COMMIT) is a community-based intervention project currently being conducted to assess the effectiveness of such community-wide strategies in increasing cessation, especially among heavy smokers [3-6].

This article describes the worksites channel in the COMMIT project. Worksites are an ideal location for promotion and support of smoking cessation efforts, including both programs and policies. Seventy percent of adults between the ages of eighteen and sixty-five are employed [7]; thus worksites provide access to large numbers of community residents who may not be reached through other means, including low income and minority groups [8, 9]. Worksites are increasingly interested in and supportive of health promotion efforts; a recent national survey of a random sample of private sector worksites with fifty or more employees indicated that 65.5 percent of worksites surveyed offered at least one type of health promotion activity [10].

Reviews of the worksite health promotion literature [11, 12], including a recent meta-analysis of worksite smoking cessation studies [13] have concluded that these smoking cessation programs have been efficacious and appear cost-effective [14]. There are several reasons for this. Multiple types of intervention can be offered repeatedly over time in worksites. By such continual contact, smokers at varying stages in the process of change–including those not yet contemplating change as well as those trying to quit–may be motivated to quit and to sustain cessation [15]. This contact may include the promotion of community-wide events or activities sponsored by other agencies. Changes in worksite norms and in the social environment, such as that which may be accomplished through nonsmoking policies, are additional supports for cessation and its maintenance [16].

In this article, we describe the COMMIT project's methods for planning interventions aimed at worksites, including the process of community analysis and the participation of the Community Board and the Worksites and Organizations Task Force. We also present the intervention protocol, standardized process objectives for this channel and strategies for tailoring the intervention protocol to the specific community. Finally, results from surveys of smokers and non-smokers in each of the intervention communities conducted early in the program are described, including information on respondents' opinions about smoking control activities in the workplace.

PLANNING FOR
COMMUNITY-BASED INTERVENTIONS

To establish initial knowledge of smoking control related activities in both the intervention and control communities, an extensive community analysis was conducted in all COMMIT communities prior to randomization. Further information to assist with intervention planning was collected in the intervention communities after randomization. For worksites, this community analysis played several important functions. Key community players and major employers were identified, including worksite leaders and providers of smoking cessation programs who were eventually invited to serve on the Community Board or the Worksites and Organizations Task Force. Using a variety of sources, we assessed community services available to worksites and identified gaps in these resources, important for program planning. We also identified "early adopter" worksites that had already made successful changes. The goal was to collect information that would allow us to understand and to compare the intervention and comparison community using nonreactive procedures, including both qualitative and quantitative approaches. Important background information was available from various printed sources, such as listings of worksites and their characteristics (e.g., size, type of industry) from the Chamber of Commerce or a state business census' newspapers and other public documents reviewing community and business concerns; and annual reports from local businesses. Interviews of community representatives provided more in-depth information. The information collected from these sources was used to tailor the intervention protocol to each of the eleven intervention communities.

The community analysis was also a means to examine the business and labor community's "culture" and history. For example, we asked: Do worksites have a history of activities or environmental changes supporting smoking cessation or other health behaviors? How extensively have the mass media covered worksite health concerns? Which health issues are of greatest priority to the business-labor community? What other community issues might divert employers' and workers' attention and energy away from health concerns? In this way the community analysis provided information on how other issues may compete with smoking control as a priority for this sector of the community. The community analysis was thus an assessment of the capability of worksites in the community to address effectively this public health problem.

Another use of the community analysis was to identify community leaders to serve on the Community Board and its various task forces. The Community Board has been involved in the overall planning of COMMIT efforts in each community; intervention activities have been planned and implemented through the task force specific to a given channel. Roles of the Community Board and its task forces have included the following [17, 18]:

1. *catalyst* for the support and involvement of community leaders;
2. *source of information* on ways to tailor the intervention to community needs;
3. *liaison* with community service providers and service vendors;
4. *clearinghouse of information* on health information, community resources and effective implementation models of health promotion;

5. *coordinator* in sponsoring community-wide health promotion activities; and

6. *support* for on-going program implementation.

The Worksites and Organizations Task Force has included representatives of the business and labor community as well as other organizations, such as churches and fraternal and civic organizations. In this article, we focus on worksites; additional intervention activities are mandated for organizations and are described elsewhere [19]. Worksites most often represented have been those already providing health promotion program or otherwise supportive of smoking control efforts. These worksites have served as pacesetters in the community and as role models for other worksites, enhancing the attractiveness of participation for other worksites [20, 21]. By working first with high profile and "early adopter" worksites it was possible to build community awareness and confidence in program efforts, thereby laying the groundwork for work with worksites less ready for change. The task force decided how to tailor the intervention protocol to the community's needs by working closely with the COMMIT project staff on the development of Annual Actions Plans, the yearly plan for accomplishing the trialwide process objectives within that community.

Goals and Assessment

The intervention was designed to support smoking cessation by changing social norms both in individual worksites and in the business community as a whole. The emphasis was on reaching large numbers of community residents through repeated interventions that together would affect social norms. Thus the COMMIT worksite plan has been guided by four intervention goals:

1. to increase smoking cessation among workers who smoke;
2. to produce changes in worksite norms to support nonsmoking;
3. to increase adoption and effective implementation of comprehensive worksite nonsmoking policies; and
4. to enhance support for nonsmoking in the business and labor sectors of the community.

The effectiveness of intervention efforts is being assessed by the extent to which specified impact objectives have been achieved. The impact objectives related to these goals for the worksite channel are presented in the top half of Table 1. Progress toward these objectives is being assessed primarily through surveys of randomly selected community residents–the evaluation cohort–and of worksites. At the worksite level, in each community thirty worksites (or a census, whichever is smaller) in each of three size strata of 50-99, 100-249, and 250 or more employees were randomly selected to be surveyed to assess level of company participation in several different types of smoking control activities, as well as worksite characteristics potentially associated with different smoking control

Table 1. Impact Objectives and Intervention Activities
for COMMIT Worksite Interventions

Impact Objectives: 1993

1. 65 percent of employed heavy smokers will report that their worksite bans smoking completely or restricts smoking to designated areas.

2. 60 percent of heavy smokers will report feeling pressure to quit smoking from co-workers.

3. 8 percent of heavy smokers will report having participated in stop smoking programs or contests and lotteries to promote cessation at their place of work.

4. 70 percent of targeted worksites will report offering lectures, classes, materials, or other programs to help or encourage employees to quit smoking within the last twelve months.

Intervention Activities

1. Smoking Policy Presentations

2. Annual Smoking Policy Workshops

3. On-Site Smoking Policy Consultations

4. Worksite Smoking Policy Network

5. Promotional Activities in the Worksite accompanying the Great American Smoke-Out, Non-Dependence Day and other Magnet Events

6. Promotion of Worksite Stop-Smoking Incentives

7. Between Worksites Challenges and Competitions

8. Dispersal of Self-Help Materials

9. Promotion of Smoker's Network

activities. These assessment procedures are described in more detail in Mattson et al. [22].

INTERVENTION PROTOCOL

The guide COMMIT project staff, the intervention protocol has defined the worksites that should be targeted in each community to increase the probability that the maximum intervention effect is achieved and that staff time is being used most effectively. In targeted worksites, at least 30 percent of employees must be community residents. Large targeted worksites have been defined as those employing 100 or more persons, while small targeted worksites employ fifty to ninety-nine persons. Intervention activities requiring significant commitment of project staff time, such as consultations on worksite policies, have been aimed at larger worksites. Smaller worksites have been targeted to assure that the high proportion of smokers employed by small worksites was included in intervention efforts. (Worksites employing less than 50 persons may be included in intervention efforts, but have not been specifically targeted given limits on staff time.)

Worksite intervention protocol activities have focused on three areas: promotion of smoking policies, motivational and incentive activities, and smoking cessation activities. For each of the nine worksite protocol activities listed in the bottom half of Table 1, standard process objectives and timelines for conducting that activity have been established to be met across all intervention communities. These process objectives establish the minimum level of activities to be conducted annually in each intervention community, as monitored by program records, a computerized data base record-keeping system.

Promotion of Smoking Policies

A growing number of worksites are adopting policies to restrict or ban smoking; according to a recent national study, a smoking policy was the most frequent type of smoking control activity engaged in by worksites [10]. Some recent studies have reported an increase in smoking cessation following a worksite's adoption of a smoking policy [23, 24], although others have found no effect on cessation but have reported a decrease in the number of cigarettes smoked at work [25-28]. The adoption of a smoking policy also may stimulate interest in participating in smoking cessation classes [24, 29, 30] and support norms conducive to cessation [31]. In the COMMIT Project, four intervention activities have promoted smoking policies, as can be seen in Table 1.

First, smoking policy presentations have been made to worksite groups such as the Chamber of Commerce or business groups on health to raise awareness about health and legal issues pertaining to smoking policies, national and local trends, and policy and program options. These presentations of at least fifteen minutes in length have been conducted during the organization's regular meetings by COMMIT project staff or by community volunteers. During the first intervention year, at least one presentation was offered in each community; in subsequent years a minimum of two presentations are being conducted annually.

Second, annual smoking policy workshops have been conducted in each intervention community, including information on smoking as a public health issue, laws and regulations, policy options and recommended procedures for implementing new policies. A smoking policy workshop guide was developed for COMMIT to assist project staff and community representatives in planning workshops [32]. Communities have adopted different strategies in presenting the annual workshop, which must be at least two to three hours in length. For example, some communities have elected to offer a workshop in conjunction with another worksite issue, such as alcohol and drug education. Others have targeted an annual workshop toward unions or small businesses. In many sites, the workshop has been co-sponsored by a local organization, such as the American Lung Association, the American Cancer Society, or the Chamber of Commerce.

Third, each intervention community has provided worksites on-site smoking policy consultations, in which information and materials have been provided to assist worksites in adopting and effectively implementing smoking policies. In some cases the needed information has been provided in a single meeting, while for other worksites multiple meetings have been necessary. For small targeted worksites, small "group" consultations with two or three worksites have been conducted. Some communities have elected to provide special training for community representatives who will be conducting these consultations. This opportunity could encourage community representatives to continue consultations once the project is terminated.

Finally, each community has established a worksite smoking policy network which lists worksites having smoking policies that are available to provide information to other worksites. This network, which is updated annually, has promoted the use of resources already existing within the community. The network has facilitated the diffusion of smoking control innovations by identifying "early adopters"–individuals and companies that have been successful in implementing a smoking ban or restrictions. A few communities were able to identify a wide assortment of businesses to put on an initial list; others either had trouble identifying places with strong policies, or–in the case of Raleigh, North Carolina, for instance–encountered reluctance regarding such publicity because of concern for repercussions from the tobacco industry. The number of companies on the first Smoking Policy Network lists ranged from just a handful (e.g., Yonkers, New York and Vallejo, California) to almost thirty (e.g., Bellingham, Washington).

Motivational and Incentive Activities

These activities were designed to encourage employees to initiate smoking cessation attempts, to maintain recent behavior changes, and to provide increased support from co-workers for cessation attempts. Incentive programs require little professional time to administer, can be used to encourage participation in educational or skills training activities, and may address issues of long term behavior change and maintenance [18]. They also can encourage those not yet ready to quit smoking to consider cessation [34]. Various types of incentives have been reported, including the use of guaranteed incentives to reinforce workers' attempts to quit for a specified time period [35, 36], contests or lottery drawings within a given worksite [37], and competitions between organizations [38, 39]. As shown in Table 1, three intervention protocol activities have used motivational and incentive strategies within the COMMIT Project.

Promotional activities have been conducted in worksites accompanying "magnet activities," such as the Great American Smoke-Out, Non-Dependent Day and other community-wide events designed to attract attention to the issue of smoking. These events have been promoted in worksites through display of materials, registration at the worksite, or accompanying events such as carbon monoxide testing. Such worksite promotions were designed to enhance the impact of community-wide events by integrating activities across channels and by increasing the likelihood of multiple exposures to a given event. Process objectives defined a cumulative increase over time in the number of worksites to be personally contacted about these events.

COMMIT has also promoted the use of motivational and incentive programs through two other protocol activities: worksite stop-smoking incentives and between-worksites challenges and competitions. The COMMIT Incentives Programs Workbook [40] has been distributed in-person to worksites to provide information about how to implement these activities. It includes guidelines on selecting awards, setting contest rules, promoting and evaluating an incentive program, and has an overall timeline and several activity planning worksheets to facilitate implementation. Consultation on the implementation of the plans has been provided on request. The workbook also provides information on between-worksite challenges and competitions, which have been facilitated by the Worksites and Organizations Task Force. During later years of the project, at least one worksite challenge or competition will be conducted each year.

Promotion of Self-Help Materials and Cessation Services

Activities and materials teaching the skills needed to quit smoking have been generally available in most communities. The COMMIT Project seeks to enhance the reach and effectiveness of these existing community services through two worksite protocol activities: distribution of self-help materials and promotion of a Smokers' Network. Self-help materials have been personally distributed by local voluntary agencies, representatives of the Smoking Cessation Resources and Services Task Force, or by COMMIT project staff to a worksite representative willing to take responsibility for the dissemination of the materials. The Smoking Cessation Resources and Services Task Force also has established a Smokers' Network, a voluntary listing of smokers in each community who receive mailings and materials to promote cessation and its maintenance. This Network has been promoted in worksites through posters, flyers, and other informational materials distributed in conjunction with promotion of community-wide and worksite events.

TAILORING THE INTERVENTION
TO THE COMMUNITY

The above intervention activities were designed to be incorporated into the community-wide intervention implementation by the COMMIT Project. By building ongoing relationships with local worksites we have been able to provide multiple and sustained interventions rather than single programs. Prior research suggests that no one treatment strategy can guarantee success; the more successful programs use multifaceted, multicomponent interventions relying on two principles: flexibility and reaching employees at various "stages of change" [41].

The intervention protocol has been tailored to each individual community by its Worksites and Organizations Task Force through the development of Annual Action Plans. Each year, this plan has described how the intervention activities will be implemented in the next year. The Annual Action Plan has outlined the tasks necessary to implement each intervention activity, identified who will conduct each task, established a timeline for completion of project tasks, and specified the resources needed to complete the tasks. The development of the Annual Action Plan has encouraged community ownership of the mandated protocol activities. Depending on the makeup of the community and the availability of resources, activities have been prioritized differently and varying community members have been involved in the implementation.

The configuration of worksites as well as cessation resources in a site has called for somewhat different priorities and activities in one community than another. Given these considerations, community boards and worksite task forces have taken advantage of the flexibility within the protocol specified activities by tailoring and localizing them in diverse ways in the Annual Action Plans and actual activities during the first two years of the four year intervention.

The Board's role has been to consider the big picture–how to increase quit rates in the community at large–and the ongoing progress of the project, and has set priorities for individual task forces accordingly. In the first two years of intervention activities, all eleven COMMIT sites endorsed the mandated worksite activities as a high priority. Some sites that did not meet all the required process objectives in the first year have assigned a greater part of their budget to worksite interventions in the second and third years, with an enhanced commitment to success in this area.

COMMIT boards and task forces also have elected to manage the mandated activities through different organizational structures. In most sites, a decision was made to hire and use COMMIT staff (e.g., a "task force coordinator" or "worksite specialist") to facilitate or carry out activities. For example, this person has often been responsible for publicity materials, dissemination of information, and negotiations with a local voluntary organization regarding the worksite smoking policy workshop. In a few sites, however, the COMMIT leadership opted to subcontract the bulk or all of an activity to a local agency. In Utica, New York, for instance, subcontracts with community agencies were set up for a "Worksite Policy Consultant" and a "Worksite Liaison" from other agencies to carry out most of the task force's directives.

As discussed above, workplaces can be ideal sites for reaching smokers, but achieving objectives in this arena has been a challenge for a number of the COMMIT communities. Thus far in the trial, some sites have found that success was not just a function of the level of effort invested. There were various reasons for this.

First, businesses were selected and contacted according to the protocol for targeting worksites, but they had to be convinced to endorse and carry out smoking control activities. Resistance may have reflected the ideas of powerful individuals in a worksite, the organizational culture, perceptions by leadership of the larger community culture as unsympathetic to smoking control activities, the potential for aggravating relations between labor and management, or merely the existence of competing priorities. Few worksites in any site have been easily recruited, and even when management cooperates fully, workers, especially heavy smokers, have not always come forth in large numbers to participate in programs. Levels of worksite involvement in COMMIT activities have varied considerably. In the first year of intervention, only a few COMMIT sites reported high participation rates–such as in Cedar Rapids, Iowa, where forty-five persons attended an initial smoking policy workshop and media coverage was provided by three television stations, the newspaper, and four radio stations. In contrast, a few sites canceled workshops for low attendance despite extensive publicity and preparation.

Second, interest in participating in COMMIT activities has varied among community business leaders and labor representatives. Task forces at some sites experienced significant turnover in membership, and have found that mobilization of community leaders for worksite endeavors must be an ongoing effort. For many business leaders who have a history of community volunteer work, smoking control was not of high priority. In many sites, potential task force members have had to be "sold" on the extent of the problem as well as on the project. In several sites, the task force had to be rebuilt after resignations and attrition of members. Turnover has occurred for many reasons; for instance, in the Ontario and North Carolina sites, several board and task force members resigned because of direct or indirect pressure due to the local tobacco industry. In other sites (e.g., Vallejo) the position of task force chair was not readily filled. The intensive early efforts of recruitment, education, and involvement of volunteers may yet yield rewards in the remaining years of the COMMIT intervention.

Finally, unlike in most prior research with worksites, those targeted for intervention activities in COMMIT ultimately are *all* those worksites in the community which satisfy the selection criteria, rather than a relatively small number picked and "cultivated" by the researchers. The scope of the COMMIT effort and the inclusiveness of its sample of larger worksites, have presented special challenges.

Past and planned COMMIT activities in the communities also have revealed creative efforts to respond to the local context. In New Mexico, community analysis showed that the business community had an unusual configuration, characterized by state government offices and a large tourist industry. The task force therefore assembled a booklet called "Santa Fe's Guide to Dining and Lodging," indicating smoking policies of restaurants and hotels. This was the only restaurant guide available in Santa Fe and has been in great demand. The New Jersey site, which stands out as one of the poorest and most ethnically diverse of the COMMIT communities, has been especially concerned about reaching blue-collar workers. A useful strategy has been to team up with other health promotion efforts in the community; carbon monoxide monitoring of smokers and ex-smokers is now being done in conjunction with blood pressure screenings provided at worksites by a local hospital. Similarly, creative approaches were needed at the Massachusetts site, where COMMIT staff encountered barriers in soliciting participation from labor groups. COMMIT staff met with representatives of several unions during a regular union meeting to make a brief presentation and to conduct a "focus group" discussion to identify ways to increase union involvement.

The Great American Smoke-Out, sponsored by the American Cancer Society, and Non-Dependence Day, sponsored by the American Lung Association, have been used successfully as vehicles for entering worksites and reaching workers. The COMMIT group in Massachusetts successfully solicited its local newspaper, the *Fitchburg Sentinel*, for a donation of eight one-quarter page ads totaling $3,000 to promote Non-Dependence Day. This was an effective way to reach smokers in the community and also reinforced collaborative efforts with the American Lung Association. Similarly, the Oregon site has had success using worksites as recruitment locations to enroll employees in a community-wide stop smoking contest and other magnet events.

COMMUNITY AND EMPLOYEE DATA
RELATED TO WORKSITE INTERVENTIONS

The communities participating in the COMMIT Project represent a diverse cross-section of communities with less than 200,000 residents. Table 2 presents general information on employees' work situations in each of the COMMIT intervention communities.

As can be seen, there were large baseline differences across communities on most variables, with the exception of percent of baseline smokers who were employed. The later data document that almost three quarters of smokers from the community could potentially be reached by worksite activities, justifying the emphasis on this intervention channel. The communities varied markedly in the number of companies with greater than 100 employees (a sevenfold difference), percent of employees working in companies with policies either prohibiting

Table 2. Worksite Related Characteristics of Intervention Communities Percentages (and Standard Error)

Intervention Community	Population[a] Age 25-64	No. Companies[b] > 100 Employees	% Smokers[c] Employed	% Employed[d] Smokers Report Restrictive Smoking Policy	% Employed[e] Smokers Report Stop Smoking Program at Work
Vallejo, CA	42759	46	69.2 (1.1)	32.9 (3.6)	28.2 (2.8)
Brantford, Ont.	38525	59	73.6 (1.2)	24.3 (3.3)	18.2 (2.2)
Cedar Rapids, IA	68749	101	76.0 (1.2)	26.0 (3.2)	40.2 (2.7)
Fitchburg/Leominster, MA	34443	68	73.9 (1.2)	12.9 (2.5)	32.2 (2.7)
Paterson, NJ	61017	68	73.9 (1.0)	24.8 (3.6)	24.2 (2.9)
Santa Fe, NM	28276	39	74.9 (0.9)	40.9 (4.0)	27.2 (2.7)
Yonkers, NY	31703	51	72.4 (1.1)	18.8 (3.1)	32.0 (2.9)
Utica, NY	38903	71	69.3 (1.2)	9.5 (2.3)	25.9 (2.6)
Raleigh, NC	81190	302	80.6 (1.0)	27.4 (3.6)	26.8 (2.5)
Medford/Ashland, OR	27441	63	70.3 (1.2)	50.9 (3.9)	27.6 (2.6)
Bellingham, WA	29795	43	66.1 (1.1)	54.6 (4.0)	26.5 (2.7)
Overall Averages	43891	83	72.7	29.4	28.1

[a] 1980 Census Data.
[b] Data from the Worksite Survey.
[c] Data from Baseline Survey.
[d] Percent of smokers reporting their worksite as having either Smokefree or Smoking Only in Designated Areas policies–Data from 1989 Evaluation Cohort Survey.
[e] Data from 1989 Evaluation Cohort Survey.

smoking or restricting it to designated areas (a fivefold difference), and availability of smoking cessation programs at work (a twofold difference). In general, there were a sizable number of moderate to large employers (≥ 100 employees) to be reached, and less than 30 percent of employees reported working in companies that had policies restricting or prohibiting smoking. Similarly, less than 30 percent of employees reported that stop smoking programs were available at their worksite.

Employees in intervention communities in the western United States were more likely to report restrictive smoking policies at their workplace than employees in other intervention communities, but this seems to be the only regional difference noted in Table 2. There appears to be either no relationship, or a modest inverse relationship, on these community level data between the percent of companies that had policies and the percent that offered cessation assistance onsite. It is also surprising that Raleigh, North Carolina, located in the heart of tobacco production, was about average on both of these factors. Additional information on worksite smoking control activities will be available after the more comprehensive surveys of employers are completed and analyzed.

Opinions of Community Members

The initial evaluation cohort survey of community members contained several attitudinal items relevant to worksite intervention. As can be seen, there was a substantial gap between public opinion about smoking policies as presented in Table 3 and the existing worksite smoking policies reported in Table 2. The overwhelming majority of smokers (80%) and almost all nonsmokers (95%) believed that environmental tobacco smoke (ETS) is harmful to a nonsmoker and that there should be bans or substantial restrictions on smoking in almost all worksites. Over 85 percent of both smokers and nonsmokers thought that smoking should be restricted or banned in both private and government workplaces. The only large difference in these data by smoking status was on preference for complete smoking bans, with 10 to 15 percent more nonsmokers than smokers supporting a complete ban. All respondent groups felt that it was more appropriate to restrict smoking in government buildings than in private workplaces.

Reaching Smokers at Work

Table 4 presents more detailed information on the work experiences of heavy (≥ 25 cigarettes per day) and light to moderate smokers. In general, there were few differences between heavy and lighter smokers on these measures. As would be expected, there were more heavy smokers among blue-collar occupations. It also is of interest that the vast majority of smokers in worksites having smoking policies felt that these policies were strictly enforced.

The most important result from the initial surveys for intervention purposes is that most smokers were employed in smaller worksites. As can be seen in Table 4,

Table 3. Worksite Smoking Related Attitudinal Items from the 1989 Evaluation Cohort Survey by Baseline Smoking Status

| Issue | Percentages (and Standard Errors) by Baseline Smoking Status | | | |
	Heavy Smokers (n = 950)[a]	Light/Moderate Smokers (n = 976)[a]	All Smokers Combined (n = 1926)[a]	Ex- and Nonsmokers (n = 2079)[a]
1. "Nonsmokers who want smoke-free air should have priority." (% agree)	52.4 (1.6)	63.2 (1.6)	57.8 (1.1)	80.8 (0.9)
2. Percent agree that ETS "is harmful to a nonsmoker."	76.5 (1.4)	83.6 (1.2)	80.1 (0.9)	95.1 (0.5)
3. Percent agreement that "smoking should be (Banned/Designated area only)" in:				
A. Government Buildings				
– Banned	8.0 (0.9)	12.3 (1.0)	10.2 (0.6)	25.3 (0.9)
– Designated area only	83.9 (1.2)	82.8 (1.2)	83.3 (0.8)	72.2 (1.0)
B. Private Workplaces				
– Banned	3.8 (0.6)	6.8 (0.8)	5.3 (0.5)	15.5 (0.8)
– Designated area only	79.5 (1.3)	82.1 (1.2)	80.8 (0.9)	78.9 (0.9)

[a] Maximum n for full sample; sample size varied slightly for each question.

Table 4. Intervention Related Characteristics of Smokers
in Intervention Communities

Question or Activity	Percentages (and Standard Errors)	
	Percent of Heavy Smokers	Percent of Light/Moderate Smokers
Which best describes your occupation?[a]		
Professional, Administrative, or Executive	33.6 (0.7)	35.0 (0.5)
Clerical, Administrative Support, Sales or Technical	24.3 (0.6)	28.7 (0.5)
Crafts, Trades, Factory Work, Service or Labor	41.2 (0.7)	35.7 (0.5)
Unclassified	0.9	0.7
How strictly are the rules for limiting smoking enforced at your place of work?[b]		
Strictly	69.1 (2.1)	69.0 (2.0)
Some	18.4 (1.8)	19.5 (1.7)
Little or No	12.6 (1.5)	11.5 (1.4)
How many people are employed where you work?[a]		
25 or Fewer	40.3 (0.7)	38.9 (0.5)
26-100	23.0 (0.6)	24.1 (0.5)
101-500	19.8 (0.6)	19.5 (0.4)
Over 500	16.9 (0.6)	17.5 (0.4)
Of those smokers who felt pressure to quit, percent reporting pressure from coworkers.[b]	41.1 (1.9)	39.4 (2.1)
Stop smoking program at work:[b]		
Aware of this activity	22.9 (1.6)	26.4 (1.6)
Participated in activity (if aware)	9.6 (2.3)	13.0 (2.4)
Stop smoking contest or lottery at work:[b]		
Aware of this activity	1.9 (0.5)	2.1 (0.5)
Participated in activity (if aware)	50.0 (13.4)	18.8 (9.8)

[a] Data from the Baseline Survey.
[b] Data from 1989 Evaluation Cohort Survey

over 60 percent of both heavy and light to moderate smokers worked at companies with 100 or fewer employees. Other analyses revealed that smaller worksites also were less likely to offer either stop-smoking programs or contests for stopping smoking. For example, employees of very small (< 25 employees), small (26-100), moderate (101-500) and large (over 500) worksites reported that 12 percent, 18 percent, 32 percent, and 56 percent, respectively, of their worksites offered stop smoking programs at work. Taken together, these data suggest that reaching smaller worksites will be an important challenge for the trial.

These data were used to refine the worksite protocol to reflect a heavier emphasis on smaller worksites. Given the limited resources, the original protocol targeted worksites with more than 100 employees. As described above, the current protocol now also specifically targets worksites having fifty to 100 employees, and sites are encouraged to the extent possible to reach even smaller worksites. To this end, a guide on worksite smoking policies was developed specifically for small businesses [33].

CONCLUSIONS

The COMMIT Project, the most extensive and costly effort to date by any government agency to increase community-wide smoking cessation rates, is an innovative project which allows researchers to assess the impact of multiple, simultaneous interventions. COMMIT also lends itself to understanding how both investigators and community leaders set priorities among approaches and develop strategies for accomplishing them.

The worksite approaches used have been shown to be effective elsewhere in more delimited research endeavors. The COMMIT approach is evaluating if these approaches can be profitably used in communities where many other smoking control activities are happening and where local people determine the specifics of "how," "where," and "by whom" they will be carried out, as well as how much of the budget to allocate to them. Initial reports from the sites, and the modification of some protocol specifications based on survey findings, have indicated a partnership between the communities and the research centers in responding to the evolving needs of the project in this key arena [3]. The data presented display differences in the eleven communities' readiness to implement smoking control activities; the pace of the eventual institutionalization of the program's goals across these communities depends in part on this initial readiness for change. The initial survey findings indicated that there is substantial opportunity for intervention in all three targeted areas–smoking policies, incentive and motivational programs, and provision of cessation resources to employees–especially in smaller worksites. Smoking control efforts through workplaces hold promise for reducing the burden of smoking in communities.

REFERENCES

1. T. F. Pechacek, *A Randomized Community Trial for Smoking Cessation*, paper presented at the 6th World Conference on Smoking and Health, Tokyo, Japan, 1987.
2. J. P. Pierce, M. C. Fiore, T. E. Novotny, E. J. Hatziandreau, and R. M. Davis, Trends in Cigarette Smoking in the U.S.–Educational Differences Are Increasing, *Journal of the American Medical Association, 261*, pp. 56-61, 1989.

3. B. Thompson, L. Wallack, E. Lichtenstein, and T. Pechacek, Principles of Community Organization and Partnership for Smoking Cessation in the Community Intervention Trial for Smoking Cessation (COMMIT), *International Quarterly of Community Health Education, 11*:3, pp. 187-203, 1990-91.

4. J. K. Ockene, E. L. Lindsay, L. Berger, and N. Hymowitz, Health Care Providers as Key Change Agents in the Community Intervention Trial for Smoking Cessation (COMMIT), *International Quarterly of Community Health Education, 11*:3, pp. 223-237, 1990-91.

5. L. Wallack and R. Sciandra, Media Advocacy and Public Education in the Community Intervention Trial for Smoking Cessation (COMMIT), *International Quarterly of Community Health Education, 11*:3, pp. 205-222, 1990-91.

6. P. Pomrehn, R. Sciandra, R. Shipley, W. Lynn, and H. Lando, Enhancing Resources for Smoking Cessation through Community Intervention: COMMIT As a Prototype, *International Journal of Community Health Education, 11*:3, pp. 259-269, 1990-91.

7. U.S. Bureau of the Census, *Statistical Abstract of the United States: 1986*, U.S. Government Printing Office, Washington, D.C., 1986.

8. P. E. Nathan, Johnson & Johnson's Live for Life: A Comprehensive Positive Lifestyle Change, in *Behavioral Health: A Handbook of Health Enhancement and Disease Prevention*, J. Matarazzo, S. Weiss, A. Herd, and N. Miller (eds.), Wiley, New York, pp. 1064-1070, 1984.

9. J. R. Terborg, The Organization as a Context for Health Promotion, in *Social Psychology and Health: The Claremont Symposium on Applied Social Psychology*, S. Oskamp and S. Spacapan (eds.), Sage Publishers, Newbury Park, California, 1988.

10. J. E. Fielding and P. V. Piserchia, Frequency of Worksite Health Promotion Activities, *American Journal of Public Health, 79*:1, pp. 16-20, 1989.

11. J. E. Fielding, Health Promotion and Disease Prevention at the Worksite, *Annual Review of Public Health, 5*, pp. 237-265, 1984.

12. R. E. Glasgow and J. Terborg, Occupational Health Promotion Programs to Reduce Cardiovascular Risk, *Journal of Consulting and Clinical Psychology, 56*, pp. 365-373, 1988.

13. K. J. Fisher, R. E. Glasgow, and J. R. Terborg, Worksite Smoking Cessation: Meta-Analysis of Long Term Quit Rates from Controlled Studies, *Journal of Occupational Medicine, 32*, pp. 429-439, 1990.

14. K. E. Warner, T. M. Wickizer, R. A. Wolfe, J. E. Schildroth, and M. H. Samuelson, Economic Implications of Workplace Health Promotion Programs: Review of the Literature, *Journal of Occupational Medicine, 30*, pp. 106-112, 1988.

15. J. S. Rossi, J. D. Prochaska, and C. C. DiClemente, Processes of Change in Heavy and Light Smokers, *Journal of Substance Abuse, 1*, pp. 1-9, 1988.

16. G. Sorensen, T. Pechacek, and U. Pallonen, Occupational and Worksite Norms and Attitudes about Smoking Cessation, *American Journal of Public Health, 76*, pp. 544-549, 1986.

17. W. M. Kizer, *The Healthy Workplace: A Blueprint for Corporate Action*, John Wiley, New York, 1987.

18. G. Sorensen, R. Glasgow, and K. Corbett, Involving Worksite and Organizations in Health Promotion, in *Organizing for Community Health Promotion: A Guide*, N. Bracht (ed.), Sage Publications, Newbury Park, California, 1990.

19. K. Corbett, et al., *The Role of Organizations in the Community Intervention Trial for Smoking Cessation*, in preparation.
20. M. A. Orlandi, The Diffusion and Adoption of Worksite Health Promotion Innovations: An Analysis of Barriers, *Preventive Medicine, 15*, pp. 522-536, 1986.
21. E. M. Rogers, *Diffusion of Innovations*, (3rd Edition), The Free Press, New York, 1983.
22. M. E. Mattson, K. M. Cummings, W. R. Lynn, C. Giffen, D. Corle, and T. Pechacek, Evaluation Plan for the Community Intervention Trial for Smoking Cessation (COMMIT), *International Quarterly of Community Health Education, 11*:3, pp. 271-290, 1990-91.
23. W. J. Millar, *Smoke in the Workplace: An Evaluation of Smoking Restrictions*, Health and Welfare Canada, Minister of Supply and Services Canada, Ottowa, 1988.
24. G. Sorensen, N. Rigotti, A. Rosen, and J. Pinney, The Effects of a Worksite Nonsmoking Policy: Evidence for Increased Cessation, *American Journal of Public Health, 81*:2, pp. 202-204, 1991.
25. L. Biener, D. B. Abrams, M. J. Follick, and L. Dean, A Comparative Evaluation of Restrictive Smoking Policy in a General Hospital, *American Journal of Public Health, 79*, pp. 192-195, 1989.
26. R. Borland, S. Chapman, N. Owen, and D. Hill, Effects of Workplace Smoking Bans on Cigarette Consumption, *American Journal of Public Health, 80*:20, pp. 172-180, 1990.
27. L. R. Petersen, S. D. Helgerson, C. M. Gibbons, C. R. Calhoun, K. H. Ciacco, and K. C. Pitchford, Employee Smoking Behavior Changes and Attitudes Following a Restrictive Policy on Worksite Smoking in a Large Company, *Public Health Reports, 103*, pp. 115-120, 1989.
28. I. M. Rosenstock, A. Stergachis, and C. Heaney, Evaluation of Smoking Prohibition Policy in a Health Maintenance Organization, *American Journal of Public Health, 76*, pp. 1014-1015, 1986.
29. M. J. Martin, Smoking Control–Policy and Legal Methods, *Western Journal of Medicine, 148*:2, p. 199, (Letter), 1988.
30. U.S. Department of Health and Human Services, *The Health Consequences of Using Smokeless Tobacco. A Report of the Surgeon General*, (DHHS Publication No. CDC 87-8398), U.S. Department of Health and Human Services, Public Health Service, Centers for Disease Control, 1986.
31. G. Sorensen and T. Pechacek, Implementing Smoking Policies in the Private Sector and Assessing Their Effects, *New York State Journal of Medicine, 89*, pp. 11-15, 1989.
32. Institute for the Study of Smoking Behavior and Policy, *COMMIT Guide to Running a Worksite Smoking Policy Workshop*, Community Intervention Trial for Smoking Cessation, National Cancer Institute, Bethesda, Maryland, 1989.
33. Institute for the Study of Smoking Behavior and Policy, *COMMIT Guide to Nonsmoking Policies for Small Businesses*, Community Interventional Trial for Smoking Cessation, National Cancer Institute, Bethesda, Maryland, 1989.
34. R. A. Winett, A. C. King, and P. G. Altman, *Health Psychology and Public Health: An Integrative Approach*, Pergamon, New York, 1989.
35. R. W Jeffrey, A. M. Pheley, J. M. Forster, M. Kramer, and N. K. Snell, Payroll Contracting for Smoking Cessation: A Worksite Pilot Study, *American Journal of Preventive Medicine, 4*, pp. 83-86, 1988.

36. D. S. Shepard and L. A. Pearlman, Health Habits that Pay Off, *Business Health*, 2, pp. 37-41, 1985.
37. S. L. Emont and K. M. Cummings, Organized Factors Affecting Participation in a Smoking Cessation Program and Abstinence among 68 Auto Dealerships, *American Journal of Health Promotion*, 5:2, pp. 107-114, 1990.
38. K. D. Brownell and M. R. J. Felix, Competitions to Facilitate Health Promotion: Review and Conceptual Analysis, *American Journal of Health Promotion*, 77, pp. 28-36, 1987.
39. R. C. Klesges, M. W. Vasey, and R. E. Glasgow, A Worksite Smoking Modification Competition: Potential for Public Health Impact, *American Journal of Public Health*, 76, pp. 198-200, 1986.
40. R. E. Glasgow and S. McRae, *Incentives Programs Workbook*, Community Intervention Trial for Smoking Cessation, National Cancer Institute, Bethesda, Maryland, 1989.
41. J. O. Prochaska and C. C. DiClemente, Stages and Processes of Self-Change of Smoking: Toward an Integrative and Model of Change, *Journal of Consulting and Clinical Psychology*, 51, pp. 390-395, 1983.

Direct reprint requests to:

Dr. Glorian Sorensen
Division of Preventive and Behavioral Medicine
University of Massachusetts Medical School
55 Lake Avenue, North
Worcester, MA 01605

ENHANCING RESOURCES FOR SMOKING CESSATION THROUGH COMMUNITY INTERVENTION: COMMIT AS A PROTOTYPE

PAUL POMREHN, M.D., M.S.
University of Iowa College of Medicine
Iowa City

RUSSELL SCIANDRA, M.S.
Roswell Park Cancer Institute
Buffalo, New York

ROBERT SHIPLEY, PH.D.
Duke University Medical School and
Veteran's Affairs Medical Center
Durham, North Carolina

WILLIAM LYNN, B.S.
National Cancer Institute
Bethesda, Maryland

HARRY LANDO, PH.D.
University of Minnesota School of Public Health
Minneapolis

For the COMMIT Research Group

ABSTRACT

Of the 17 million smokers in North America who attempt to quit smoking each year, fewer than one in ten succeed [1, 2]. How can communities improve smokers' chances of quitting? The National Cancer Institute addresses this question through COMMIT, the Community Intervention Trial for Smoking Cessation. COMMIT is the largest smoking intervention trial in the world, involving over 2 million people in twenty-two North

Int'l. Quarterly of Community Health Education, Vol. 11(3) 259-269, 1990-91

© 1991, Baywood Publishing Co., Inc.

American communities. The study protocol requires that the implementation of mandated interventions in each community be managed by a Community Board and at least four task forces (Health Care, Worksites and Organizations, Cessation Resources, and Public Education, including Media and Youth). Three required and three optional interventions in the COMMIT protocol relate to the availability of cessation resources and services. The Cessation Resources Task Force, composed of community volunteers, supervises implementation of these interventions at each site. The activities of each task force are integrated with the others in a community action plan. How COMMIT activities enhance the utilization of cessation resources and services and how these services fit into a community intervention is the subject of this article. Descriptions of the study design and evaluation plan, and of the community mobilization process are presented elsewhere [3, 4].

THE AVAILABILITY AND USE OF
CESSATION RESOURCES

Cessation resources includes the broad range of existing materials and methods designed to encourage or help people to quit smoking. The spectrum includes educational or self-help materials, in multiple formats such as pamphlets, books, audio and video tapes and even microprocessors; lectures; support services like smoking hotlines or information services; and group and individual treatment programs.

A wealth of knowledge exists regarding methods and techniques that can aid smokers who are trying to quit [5-8]. In *Reducing the Health Consequences of Smoking: 25 Years of Progress*, the U.S. Surgeon General reports that specific strategies for helping people stop smoking have not changed much over the past twenty-five years. However, how strategies are packaged and marketed to reach groups with high smoking prevalence has improved [1]. Nearly all types of cessation interventions utilize self-help materials and strategies in some form.

The Surgeon General's review of cessation methods used in the last twenty-five years summarized the follow-up quit rates of 416 smoking cessation trials by intervention method. The twenty-two intervention categories included self-help and education interventions, group programs, physician interventions, acupuncture, hypnosis, etc. Regardless of interventions, most smokers return to smoking within one year. The Report concludes that variation in success within and between methods was most likely attributable to differences in the way smokers select or were selected into various programs, not because of inherent superiority of any particular method [1].

Cessation resources are provided by a number of organizations. Historically, the American Cancer Society, the American Lung Association and the American Heart Association have been the major providers of cessation services and self-help materials [1]. Local hospitals and other community service agencies also offer a broad spectrum of cessation services. Most of these organizations offer quality services at very reasonable cost.

In spite of the availability of many types and sources of assistance, smokers prefer quitting on their own [5]. The 1986 Adult Use of Tobacco Survey demonstrates that 90 percent of successful quitters quit without participating in an "assisted method" such as program/course, hypnosis, psychological/psychiatric services, or nicotine gum prescription [9]. The low utilization of assisted methods has prompted some to argue the cessation clinics be abandoned [10]. Altman et al., after demonstrating that cessation clinics are not as cost-effective as self-help approaches or quitting contests, argue that combined cessation approaches may increase effectiveness and provide options that appeal to a wider variety of smokers [11].

With this evidence in mind, COMMIT investigators made several important assumptions that influenced protocol development: 1) A wide variety of services and resources are generally available in communities through existing agencies; it was not necessary to develop new cessation services as part of COMMIT. 2) Evidence does not support favoring one cessation method over others, hence the individual smoker is probably the best judge of which method meets his or her needs. 3) Since 90 percent of smokers prefer to quit on their own; providing motivation and improving their access to self-help materials appears to be the most promising intervention strategy.

THE COMMIT APPROACH TO CESSATION RESOURCES

A fundamental assumption underlying the COMMIT intervention is that essential to increasing cessation rates is change in the social circumstances surrounding smokers' decisions to quit, to initiate quitting, and to maintain abstinence. Thus, project resources are directed toward generating peer group influence and social support for cessation with the expectation that the supply of cessation services will expand as needed to meet the increased demand created by COMMIT. Activities aimed at enhancing access to self-help cessation materials and raising awareness of services are integrated into the protocol mandates of each task force [12, 13]. Activities of the Cessation Resources Task Force are directed primarily towards distributing information to prospective quitters. The impact objectives and required and optional activities for the task force are shown in Table 1.

Develop and Maintain a Cessation Resources Guide

Fiore et al. discuss several barriers that inhibit utilization of cessation resources [9]. Because of timing, location, and expense, some resources are inaccessible to smokers when they need them. Also smokers may be unaware of all available resources in their community.

The COMMIT protocol requires the publication and distribution of smoking cessation resource guides. Resource guides are community specific, non-evaluative descriptions of local cessation resources. The guides list organizations

Table 1. Cessation Resources Task Force Objectives
and Intervention Activities

Impact Objectives

1. By 1993, 80% of smokers will be aware of the availability of stop-smoking programs or classes in their community as measured in the evaluation cohort survey.
2. By 1993, cessation materials will be distributed to the equivalent of 20% of smokers as measured by the cessation resources survey.
3. By 1993, cessation clinics will have been attended by the equivalent of 8% of smokers as measured by the cessation resources survey.
4. By 1993, the Smokers Network will have enrolled 8% of heavy smokers as measured by program records.

Activities

Required

1. Develop and Maintain a Cessation Resources Guide.
2. Recruit Heavy Smokers Into the Smokers' Network Through Hotline, Magnet Events and Youth Activities.
3. Prepare and Distribute a Semi-Annual Newsletter.

Optional

1. Special Recruitment Activities.
2. Symposium on Smoking Cessation.
3. Utilize Existing Hotlines.

or individuals that offer smoking cessation programs, sources of self-help materials and cessation aids. A brief description of each service includes names and telephone numbers of contact persons.

All eleven COMMIT intervention communities have produced a resource guide. Content and format were developed locally, and decisions about which services to list were left to each community. In general, listing has been inclusive rather than exclusive–providing consumers with as many options as possible. Little or no controversy has arisen in the communities about the content of the guides. Many were formatted as a 3 ö 8 pamphlet that unfolds into a small poster for display on a bulletin board. They often include motivational material to encourage smokers to quit, such as a self-administered questionnaire on nicotine addiction.

Distribution channels for the guide are determined at the local level. Guides have been distributed widely through physicians' and dentists' offices, clinics, hospitals, worksites, point of purchase displays in retail outlets such as pharmacies, at health fairs, and as part of self-help packets distributed during community events such as the Great American Smokeout. At the Brantford, Ontario site, resource guides were distributed to every household in the community through a direct mail advertising packet. In Medford/Ashland, Oregon, distribution was accomplished primarily through worksites and health care provider offices. By these means, 20,000 guides have been distributed in the first two years of intervention.

Recruit Heavy Smokers into the Smokers' Network

Quitting smoking is a process that involves several stages [14, 15]. Individuals often go through the stages of quitting several times before they achieve long-term success. The broad range of activities offered in COMMIT communities are designed to stimulate quitting in thousands of smokers. Maintaining communication with smokers who attempt to quit is an opportunity to prevent relapse or to encourage relapsers to try again.

The Smokers' Network serves primarily as the newsletter mailing list. Its success depends on the recruitment of smokers through many channels. The Cessation Resources and Services Task Force coordinates strategies to recruit heavy smokers to join the Network.

Smokers voluntarily join the Network by participating in activities such as community-wide "Quit and Win" promotions. Both the Medford/Ashland, Oregon and Raleigh, North Carolina sites used cards to sign up contestants and enroll them in the Network. Several other sites have used community-wide events as opportunities to build their Network mailing lists. In Vallejo, California, COMMIT has produced a stand-up display entitled "I'd Like to Quit But I Think I Need Help." Attached is a pad of tear-off Network sign-up forms. The Yonkers, New York site has developed a similar poster for worksites. When feasible, cessation activities in worksites and organizations promoting smoking cessation have included information on the availability of the Network and provided opportunities for smokers to voluntarily enroll. For example, Network sign-up cards are made available when carbon monoxide testing is done during worksite promotion in the Raleigh site. Although physician and dentist training sessions include information about the Smokers Network, as yet health care providers have not been a major source of Network referrals.

In many sites, Network mailing lists have grown more slowly than anticipated. Presently, only the Oregon site has exceeded the objective of signing up 10 percent of smokers to their Network. Many sites have enrolled only 200-400 Network members. Network recruitment strategies are being re-examined in many sites to increase enrollment. Asking smokers to complete, sign, and return a Network card apparently creates too many barriers to participation.

Prepare and Distribute a Semi-Annual Newsletter

All sites are required to produce and distribute a newsletter at least twice a year. The newsletters, intended primarily for smokers, are supportive and sensitive to their needs. Each edition contains community-specific information, a calendar of events related to smoking cessation, and instructions on how to sign up to receive the newsletter. Regular features have included stories on local celebrities or representative smokers who succeeded in quitting smoking, tips on quitting smoking on one's own, humorous stories about smoking, interesting facts about smoking and its health effects, and descriptions of upcoming special events of interest to smokers.

Field staff have been responsible for writing copy and selecting materials in most sites, while some have relied on an editorial board composed of staff and task force members. For the most part, newsletters have been printed locally. Initial newsletter editions have been distributed through worksites, physicians, and dentists, offices, health fairs, self-help "quit kits" and by mail. In Raleigh and Vallejo, newsletters were delivered to all households in the community through occupant mailings. The Smokers' Network mailing lists, though growing, have only a few hundred names at most sites and are not yet a major means of newsletter distribution.

Like the resource guides, the newsletter is a useful small medium for information diffusion. Wide distribution is assisting growth of the Network. Network sign-up cards, which are attached to the newsletter, have been returned by over 200 recipients in Raleigh. Response to the newsletter in Cedar Rapids has been positive–so much so that the Community Board and staff decided to publish one every two months. There, newsletters are distributed by hospital courier to every physician's office where they are made available to patients in the waiting room.

Optional Cessation Resources Activities

The COMMIT protocol includes several optional activities which may be undertaken if resources permit.

Special Recruitment Activities

Heavy smokers have not been as successful at quitting as light-moderate smokers [1]. In fact, heavy smokers are less likely to have tried to quit smoking [16]. Recognizing that reaching heavy smokers may require additional approaches not specifically described in the protocol, this optional activity encourages each COMMIT community to think about how to reach heavy smokers and to customize plans to fit each community's unique situation.

Paterson, New Jersey, an urban site with a high proportion of African-American residents, uses an existing network of well attended hypertension screening clinics to reach the black community. Information about smoking, smoking cessation, and COMMIT activities is distributed at screening sites. The Utica, New York site used a similar approach to reach over 20,000 individuals, over 20 percent of them smokers.

Utica and Cedar Rapids, Iowa have developed marketing plans to reach smokers using radio and television spots and billboards. Smokers are instructed to call the COMMIT field offices for information. These campaigns are stimulating five to six calls per day from smokers requesting information.

Symposium on Smoking Cessation

Providers of cessation services share a common interest in recruiting smokers and helping smokers succeed in quitting. Sites may conduct an educational meeting for providers to stimulate interaction and keep them abreast of new developments in cessation. Since COMMIT activities are likely to increase the demand for cessation services, discussion of how providers will meet the demand will also be relevant. Some sites have conducted a symposium, while others report no interest among providers in such an activity.

Medford/Ashland, Oregon attracted over fifty participants to a half-day symposium just prior to the Great American Smokeout. Many attendees were student nurses whose interest was stimulated by problems in dealing with patients who were pressuring them for cigarettes in a hospital that had recently gone smoke-free. COMMIT played a facilitative role in changing the hospital's policy. This was an example of how an environmental change increases the salience of the smoking issue and interacts with cessation services.

Utilize Existing Regional Hotline

A telephone hotline provides smokers easy access to information on cessation, brief counseling, and referral assistance [17]. The experience of the National Cancer Institute's Cancer Information Service (CIS) has shown high utilization rates by heavy smokers when advertising promotes the number as a source of smoking cessation advice [18, 19].

In addition to personal counseling of callers, the hotline may provide information and referral to cessation services. Hotlines have been effectively used in conjunction with quit-smoking magnet events, such as a newspaper smoking cessation series [19].

The funding available to COMMIT sites does not include an allocation for a dedicated hotline. Hotlines are labor-intensive and given the relatively small populations of the intervention communities, dedicated hotlines may not be cost-effective. Therefore, sites have been urged to independently establish working relationships with regional hotlines such as the CIS, the American Cancer Society's Cancer Response System or the American Lung Association's Freedom Line.

Hotlines may serve several functions in COMMIT. In addition to personal counseling of callers, the hotline may provide information and referral to cessation

Table 2. Availability of Cessation Resources in COMMIT Communities: Median Number of Providers Offering Services by Provider Type and Service

	Provider		
Services	Voluntary Agency	Hospital	Proprietary Program
Materials distribution	5 (2-8)[a]	2 (0-4)	2 (0-11)
Cessation classes	2 (0-3)	2 (0-3)	3 (0-14)
Informational talks	3 (0-6)	1 (0-3)	1 (0-7)
Worksite assistance	2 (0-6)	1 (0-3)	0 (0-5)

[a] Median with range in parentheses.

services. Hotlines have been effectively used in conjunction with quit- smoking magnet events, such as a newspaper smoking cessation series [20].

Hotline interventions have been used at some COMMIT sites. Most sites list the CIS number (1-800-4-CANCER) in their resource guide. Some sites have used other existing hotlines. The Oregon site used the American Lung Association "Freedom Line" to provide information about their "Quit and Win" contest. Cedar Rapids used a recorded message with a voice mailbox (Cityline) to support a television cessation series. Over 800 calls came to Cityline during the quit series, with 350 callers leaving their name and address so self-help materials could be sent to them.

DISCUSSION

Most smokers quit on their own. Cohen and others reported on ten prospective studies of self-initiated quitting with and without self-help materials [21]. After twelve months follow-up, about 14 percent were abstinent [21]. Self-help approaches are more appealing to smokers and most cost effective. Clinic programs are also effective and may appeal to some smokers who cannot quit on their own [7, 8].

Since the COMMIT protocol was developed, several pertinent surveys have been completed in the study communities. These surveys provide an opportunity to re-examine the assumptions that guided cessation resource related activities. We know from a systematic survey in all twenty-two COMMIT communities that the major voluntary agencies distribute information about smoking and offer cessation classes in various settings (Table 2). Hospital and proprietary cessation services are also readily available in COMMIT communities. Capacity to provide services to worksites needs to be increased in some communities. In general, as shown in Table 2, the assumption that most needed resources already exist was accurate.

Do current smokers intend to use available resources? The Evaluation Cohort survey conducted between January and April of 1989, asked current smokers in

Table 3. Percentage of Ex-Smokers Using Each Type of Assistance During Their Last Year as Smokers: All Communities Combined[a]

Type of Assistance[b]	Males (Ages)		Females (Ages)		All
	25-44 (N = 1288)	45-64 (N = 767)	25-44 (N = 1368)	45-64 (N = 599)	(N = 4022)
Help from doctor/dentist	7.6	14.2	8.8	12.4	10.0
Nicorette gum	7.8	12.5	7.9	10.7	9.2
Quit with other smokers	18.7	14.6	10.3	15.5	18.0
Thru prayer/religious reasons	9.9	9.1	12.6	13.7	11.2
Cutting down amount smoked	28.2	22.4	29.2	20.0	26.2
Quit cold turkey	90.3	90.0	88.6	86.1	89.0
Local health agency	3.2	6.3	5.6	5.8	5.0
Used a commercial program	2.1	3.9	2.6	3.5	2.8
Program offered thru work	2.6	2.5	2.4	3.2	2.6
Read books, pamphlets, etc.	10.6	10.0	12.4	10.2	11.1
Used advice thru media/radio/TV	15.2	11.2	13.3	13.0	13.5
Used toll-free # for information	0.8	1.3	0.0	0.5	0.9
Participated in a community event	6.8	6.3	7.7	5.3	6.8

[a] Respondents were allowed more than one answer, therefore, percentages total more than 100 percent.
[b] Items listed in order they were presented by interviewers.

the eleven COMMIT intervention communities, "If you wanted to quit smoking what local person or organization would you contact for information about stopping smoking?" [4]. Of the 1,506 smokers interviewed, less than half were able to identify a source of help: 21.4 percent said they would contact their doctor, 20.5 percent would contact a voluntary health agency such as the American Cancer Society, American Lung Association or American Heart Association and 8.3 percent would contact a local hospital or health department. Only 23 percent of smokers knew there is a toll-free number to call for information about stopping smoking, and 54 percent said they knew of local stop-smoking programs.

Do smokers use available resources when they quit? Over 4,000 persons who had successfully quit smoking within the five years prior to their interview were asked what type of assistance they had in the year they successfully quit. These data are summarized in Table 3. (Respondents could name more than one means of assistance.) Eighty-nine percent indicated they stopped "cold turkey or just quit." However, successful quitters, even those who say they "just quit," often report receiving assistance from doctors and dentists, other smokers, ministers, health agencies and the mass media. Only about one in ten successful ex-smokers used formal programs. A similar proportion used self-help materials.

Ex-smokers in COMMIT communities quit on their own without much formal assistance. These results are very similar to those reported by Fiore [9], and support the notion that COMMIT resources should be directed towards increasing awareness and utilization of existing services while enhancing the availability of self-help materials.

COMMIT is taking a broad spectrum approach to enhancing the use of cessation resources. The protocol anticipates that thousands of persons will be making attempts to quit smoking during the course of the trial. Communities have a wide variety of available resources–from intensive clinic programs to informational flyers. With regard to cessation resources, the COMMIT intervention will enhance awareness of those resources and encourage smokers to choose cessation services based on their individual preference. By integrating information about existing resources with as many COMMIT activities as possible, e.g., in worksites, health facilities, magnet events and in the media, COMMIT will increase utilization of cessation resources and services. We believe this strategy will result in increased quit rates in the eleven intervention communities.

REFERENCES

1. U.S. Department of Health and Human Services, *Reducing the Health Consequences of Smoking: 25 Years of Progress. A Report of the Surgeon General*, U.S. Department of Health and Human Services, Public Health Service, Centers for Disease Control, Center for Chronic Disease Prevention and Health Promotion, Office on Smoking and Health, DHHS Publication No. (CDC) 89-8411, 1989.
2. E. J. Hatziandreu, J. P. Pierce, M. Lefkopoulou, et al., Quitting Smoking in the United States in 1986, *Journal of the National Cancer Institute*, in press.
3. B. Thompson, L. Wallack, E. Lichtenstein, and T. Pechacek, Principles of Community Organization and Partnership for Smoking Cessation in the Community Intervention Trial for Smoking Cessation (COMMIT), *International Quarterly of Community Health Education, 11*:3, pp. 187-203, 1990-91.
4. M. E. Mattson, K. M. Cummings, W. R. Lynn, C. Giffen, D. Corle, and T. Pechacek, Evaluation Plan for the Community Intervention Trial for Smoking Cessation (COMMIT), *International Quarterly of Community Health Education, 11*:3, pp. 271-290, 1990-91.
5. J. L. Schwartz, A Critical Review and Evaluation of Smoking Control Methods, *Public Health Reports, 84*, pp. 483-506, 1969.
6. J. L. Schwartz and G. Rider, *Review and Evaluation of Smoking Control Methods: United States and Canada, 1969-1977*, U.S. Department of Health, Education and Welfare, Bethesda, Maryland, HEW Publication (CDC) 79-8369, 1978.
7. J. L. Schwartz, *Review and Evaluation of Smoking Cessation Methods: United States and Canada, 1978-1985*, U.S. Department of Health and Human Services, National Institutes of Health Publication 87-2940, 1987.
8. R. E. Glasgow and E. Lichtenstein, Long-Term Effects of Behavioral Smoking Cessation Interventions, *Behavior Therapy, 18*, pp. 297-324, 1987.
9. M. C. Fiore, T. E. Novotny, J. P. Pierce, G. A. Giovino, E. J. Hatziandreu, P. A. Newcomb, T. S. Surawicz, and R. M. Davis, Methods Used to Quit Smoking in the

United States: Do Cessation Programs Help?, *Journal of the American Medical Association, 263*:20, pp. 2760-2765, 1990.

10. S. Chapman, Stop-Smoking Clinics: A Case for Their Abandonment, *The Lancet*, pp. 918-920, April 20, 1985.

11. D. G. Altman, J. A. Flora, S. P. Fortmann, and J. W. Farquhar, The Cost-Effectiveness of Three Smoking Cessation Programs, *American Journal of Public Health, 77*, pp. 162-165, 1987.

12. J. K. Ockene, E. L. Lindsay, L. Berger, and N. Hymowitz, Health Care Providers as Key Change Agents in the Community Intervention Trial for Smoking Cessation (COMMIT), *International Quarterly of Community Health Education, 11*:3, pp. 223-237, 1990-91.

13. G. Sorensen, R. E. Glasgow, and K. Corbett, Promoting Smoking Control through Worksites in the Community Intervention Trial for Smoking Cessation (COMMIT), *International Quarterly of Community Health Education, 11*:3, pp. 239-257, 1990-91.

14. J. O. Prochaska and C. C. DiClemente, Stages and Processes of Self-Change of Smoking: Toward an Integrative Model of Change, *Journal of Consulting and Clinical Psychology, 51*, pp. 390-395, 1983.

15. T. J. Rosen and R. H. Shipley, A Stage Analysis of Self-Initiated Smoking Reductions, *Addictive Behaviors, 8*, pp. 263-272, 1983.

16. U.S. Department of Health and Human Services, *The Health Benefits of Quitting*, Department of Health and Human Services, Public Health Service, Centers for Disease Control, Office on Smoking and Health, 1990, in press.

17. J. A. Ward, K. Duffy, R. Sciandra, and S. Karlins, What the Public Wants to Know about Cancer: The Cancer Information Service, *The Cancer Bulletin, 40*, pp. 384-389, 1988.

18. C. R. Jaen, K. M. Cummings, S. L. Emont, and R. Sciandra, Promotion of a Stop Smoking Telephone Information and Referral Service, *Advances in Health Education: Current Research*, in press.

19. K. M. Cummings, R. Sciandra, S. Davis, and B. Rimer, Response to an Anti-Smoking Campaign Aimed at Mothers with Young Children, *Health Education Research: Theory & Practice, 4*, pp. 429-437, 1989.

20. K. M. Cummings, R. Sciandra, and S. Markello, Impact of a Newspaper-Mediated Quit Smoking Program, *American Journal of Public Health*, November 1987.

21. S. Cohen, E. Lichtenstein, J. O. Prochaska, J. S. Rossi, E. R. Gritz, C. R. Carr, C. T. Orleans, V. J. Schoenbach, L. Biener, D. Abrams, C. DiClemente, S. Curry, G. A Marlatt, K. M. Cummings, S. L. Emont, G. Giovino, and D. Ossip-Klein, Debunking Myths about Self-Quitting: Evidence from Ten Prospective Studies of Persons Quitting Smoking by Themselves, *American Psychologist, 44*, pp. 1355-1365, 1989.

Direct reprint requests to:

Paul Pomrehn, M.D.
Department of Preventive Medicine
2812 Steindler Building
University of Iowa
Iowa City, IA 52242

EVALUATION PLAN FOR THE COMMUNITY INTERVENTION TRIAL FOR SMOKING CESSATION (COMMIT)

MARGARET E. MATTSON, PH.D.
National Cancer Institute
Bethesda, Maryland

K. MICHAEL CUMMINGS, PH.D., M.P.H.
Roswell Park Memorial Institute
Buffalo, New York

WILLIAM R. LYNN, B.S.
National Cancer Institute, Bethesda, Maryland

CAROL GIFFEN, D.V.M.
IMS
Silver Spring, Maryland

DON CORLE, M.S.

TERRY PECHACEK, PH.D.

National Cancer Institute
Bethesda, Maryland

For the COMMIT Research Group

ABSTRACT

The National Cancer Institute is sponsoring the Community Intervention Trial for Smoking Cessation (COMMIT), a multi-center research project designed to test the value of a community-based effort to promote smoking cessation. The trial involves eleven matched pairs of communities with random assignment of one community per pair to the intervention or to the comparison

Int'l. Quarterly of Community Health Education, Vol. 11(3) 271-290, 1990-91

© 1991, Baywood Publishing Co., Inc.

condition. This article reviews the rationale and methodology of the COM-MIT evaluation plan which is organized into four components: 1) *outcome assessment*, monitoring changes in community smoking patterns; 2) *impact assessment*, measuring the effect of the COMMIT intervention on mediating factors thought to be important in facilitating changes in community smoking behavior (e.g., social norms supporting nonsmoking); 3) *process assessment*, monitoring the quality and timeliness of intervention delivery; and 4) *economic assessment*, estimating the cost effectiveness of the intervention.

The National Cancer Institute (NCI) has identified a rapid reduction in the national prevalence of adult smoking as a primary objective in its goal to reduce cancer mortality rates by 50 percent by the year 2000 [1]. Because heavy smokers often have the greatest difficulty quitting and account for the largest proportion of deaths due to smoking [1, 2], they have been targeted for special attention by the NCI's Community Intervention Trial for Smoking Cessation (COMMIT). The purpose of COMMIT is to test a community based intervention approach to smoking control.

This article reviews the rationale and methodology of the COMMIT evaluation plan. The goal of the plan is to measure changes in community smoking patterns associated with COMMIT and to allow testing of the assumptions which have guided the development of intervention strategies. The evaluation plan is organized into four components: 1) *outcome evaluation*, which measures changes in smoking behavior; 2) *impact evaluation*, which measures changes in factors thought to be important in facilitating community wide smoking behavior changes (e.g., social norms about smoking, tobacco intervention activities by health care providers, media coverage of tobacco issues); 3) *process evaluation*, which documents the adequacy of intervention implementation; and 4) *economic evaluation*, which will estimate the cost effectiveness of the COMMIT intervention.

TRIAL OVERVIEW AND STUDY DESIGN

COMMIT is a multi-center experiment designed to test a community-based strategy to promote smoking cessation in persons who smoke twenty-five or more cigarettes per day [3]. The project involves eleven research centers (plus a Coordination Center) and twenty-two communities in North America. Each research center participating in the trial is responsible for one intervention and one comparison community. Communities participating in the trial vary in population size from approximately 54,000 to 167,000. For the purposes of the trial, a community was broadly defined to include an individual city, multiple smaller cities geographically linked, and portions of well-defined metropolitan areas.

Research centers selected communities which were matched, to the degree feasible, on variables known or believed to influence smoking cessation rates. Matching characteristics included community size, demographic profile, mobility/migration patterns, smoking prevalence, health care and media

Table 1. Research Centers and the 11 Community Pairs
Participating in COMMIT

Research Centers	Community Pairs (I/C)*	Population Size	Smoking Prevalence**
American Health Foundation	Yonkers (I)	63,278	29.4%
New York, New York	New Rochelle (C)	57,493	28.9
Fred Hutchinson Cancer Center	Bellingham (I)	65,632	23.9
Seattle, Washington	Longview/Kelso (C)	60,424	28.5
Kaiser Foundation Research Institute	Vallejo (I)	89,046	28.7
Oakland, California	Hayward (C)	121,134	28.0
Lovelace Medical Foundation	Santa Fe (I)	57,572	23.2
Albuquerque, New Mexico	Las Cruces (C)	53,757	22.6
New Jersey University of Medicine and Dentistry	Paterson (I)	138,317	31.3
Newark, New Jersey	Trenton (C)	91,726	34.7
Oregon Research Institute	Medford/Ashland (I)	58,929	24.5
Eugene, Oregon	Albany/Corvallis (C)	73,452	23.1
Research Triangle Institute	Raleigh (I)	163,036	24.9
Research Triangle, North Carolina	Greensboro (C)	166,824	29.3
Roswell Park Cancer Institute	Utica (I)	85,490	32.4
Buffalo, New York	Binghamton/Johnson City (C)	76,418	31.4
University of Iowa	Cedar Rapids (I)	144,835	26.8
Iowa City, Iowa	Davenport (C)	136,408	29.1
University of Massachusetts Medical School	Fitchburg/Leominster (I)	75,805	31.2
Worcester, Massachusetts	Lowell (C)	92,418	33.7
Waterloo Research Institute	Brantford (I)	86,985	35.2
Waterloo, Ontario Canada	Peterborough (C)	84,800	33.7

* I = Intervention community; C = Comparison community.
** Smoking prevalence estimates are based on the baseline survey of adult smokers between the ages of 25-64 years conducted in 1988.

resources. Table 1 lists the research centers and the eleven community pairs participating in COMMIT.

The trial began in September 1986 and will end in December 1994. The project is being implemented in three phases. In Phase 1 (October 1986 to October 1988), project investigators worked together to develop a standard intervention protocol and an evaluation plan, and to conduct baseline assessments in the eleven paired communities. In the current Phase 2 (October 1988 to June 1993), the intervention protocol is being implemented in the eleven designated experimental communities. The specific intervention strategies for COMMIT have been described elsewhere [4-8]. In early 1993, final outcome assessments will be conducted to measure the impact of the four years of intervention. During Phase 3 (July 1993 to December 1994), the investigators will analyze the results of the trial and prepare trial reports summarizing findings.

Allocation to experimental and comparison conditions within a community pair was done by randomization in May 1988, after completion of a baseline survey to measure smoking prevalence and identify cohorts of smokers. Results from the baseline survey and from background information collected prior to randomization show that the community pairs are comparable with respect to demographics, smoking prevalence, and community resources (e.g., hospitals, media outlets).

The primary hypothesis being tested in COMMIT is that the implementation of a defined protocol, delivered through multiple community groups and organizations and using limited external resources, will result in a quit rate among heavy smokers that is at least ten percentage points greater (e.g., 25% versus 15%) than the quit rate observed among heavy smokers in the comparison communities. The evaluation plan will assess multiple indicators of the impact of the intervention. However, the primary measure of the trial's success is based upon the quit rate in a representative sample of heavy smokers. The sample size and statistical considerations of the trial are described by Byar et al. [9].

OUTCOME EVALUATION

Outcome evaluation is designed to measure the effect of the COMMIT intervention on: 1) smoking cessation rates among cohorts of heavy smokers; 2) smoking cessation rates among cohorts of light to moderate smokers; 3) the prevalence of overall smoking among adults; and 4) smoking onset among adolescents. See Table 2 for a summary of the main features of the prevalence, endpoint cohort, evaluation cohort and adolescent surveys, each of which will be discussed below.

The primary outcome measure in the trial is the smoking cessation rate of a representative cohort of heavy smokers. A heavy smoker is defined as a current smoker of twenty-five or more cigarettes per day. A secondary outcome measure in the trial is the smoking cessation rate of a representative cohort of light and moderate smokers. Light and moderate smokers include current smokers of fewer than twenty-five cigarettes daily. Cohorts of heavy and light/moderate smokers in all twenty-two communities were selected from among current smokers identified in a baseline survey conducted in 1988.

Prevalence Surveys

Between January and April 1988, a survey of approximately 6,000 households in each of the twenty-two communities were conducted. This telephone survey was conducted centrally by two commercial survey research companies. Modified

Table 2. Major Features of COMMIT Surveys

Survey	Objectives	Data Collection Method	Year(s)	Sample Size	Content of Survey
Baseline	- Estimate prevalence - Identify smoker cohorts	- Centrally conducted telephone survey	1988	- 6000 households per community	- Smoking history - Smoking status of household members - Demographics - Cohort tracking information
Endpoint cohort	- Estimate cessation rate in heavy, light/moderate cohorts identified in baseline survey	- Centrally conducted telephone survey	1989-93 (annually)	- 400 heavy smokers per community - 400 light/moderate smokers per community	- Current cigarette smoking status
Final prevalence	- Estimate smoking prevalence - Measure attitudes about smoking	- Centrally conducted telephone survey	1993	- 1500 households per community	- Smoking status of household members - Attitudes/beliefs re tobacco use - Demographics - Exposure to Smoking Control activities (e.g., media, at work)

275

Table 2. (Cont'd.)

Survey	Objectives	Data Collection Method	Year(s)	Sample Size	Content of Survey
Youth	- Estimate tobacco use habits of adolescents - Measure attitudes about tobacco use	- Locally conducted classroom survey of ninth grade students	1990 1993	- 450 students per community	- Current and past tobacco use - Attitudes/beliefs re tobacco use - Exposure to tobacco prevention information at school, in media
Evaluation cohort	- Measure knowledge and attitudes about tobacco use - Measure exposure to smoking control activities delivered via media, at work, from health care providers	- Centrally conducted telephone survey	1989 1991 1993	-100 heavy smokers -100 light/moderate smokers -100 recent ex-smokers -100 nonsmokers (per community)	- Knowledge of dangers of smoking - Beliefs about benefits of stopping - Attitudes about restricting smoking - Exposure to smoking control activities (e.g., media, worksite
Health care provider	- Measure physician and dentist tobacco counseling practices	- Centrally conducted mailed survey of physicians and dentists	1990a 1993	- All primary care physicians and general practice dentists	- Tobacco counseling practices (e.g., advice, distribution of cessation materials)

Setting	Objectives	Method	Year	Sample	Measures
Health care offices	- Estimate prevalence of smokfree facilities - Assess availability of cessation resources	- Locally conducted telephone survey of physician and dental offices	1990a 1993	- Random sample of 30 private physicians and 30 dental offices per community	- Presence/type of smoking policy - Availability of tobacco education materials (e.g., posters, pamphlets) - Office characteristics (e.g., number of staff)
Worksites	- Estimate prevalence of smokefree worksites - Assess availability of cessation assistance for employees	- Centrally conducted telephone survey	1990a 1993	- Random sample of 30 worksites with 50-99 employees, 30 worksites with 100-249 employees, and 30 worksites with 250 or more employees per community. All schools included in frame.	- Presence/type of smoking policy - Availability/type of cessation services for employees (e.g., clinics, incentives) - Worksite characteristics (e.g., type of business, union)
Religious organizations	- Estimate prevalence of smokefree religious organizations	- Centrally conducted telephone survey	1990a 1993	- Random sample of 50 churches or synagogues per community	- Presence/type of smoking policy - Availability/type of cessation services for members - Characteristics of organization (i.e., number of members)

Table 2. (Cont'd.)

Survey	Objectives	Data Collection Method	Year(s)	Sample Size	Content of Survey
Cessation resources	- Estimate number of local agencies providing smoking control services - Assess type and quantity of cessation services available in the community	- Locally conducted telephone survey	1989 1991 1993	- All of following agencies within a community: voluntary agencies, hospitals, health departments, HMO's, medical/ dental societies, libraries, proprietary program	- Type of services provided (e.g., cessation classes, pamphlets, information talks, worksite consultations) - Frequency and use of service - Characteristics of agency

Note: a = intervention community only;
all other surveys conducted in both intervention and comparison sites.

random digit dialing and geographic boundary screening were used to obtain representative samples of households within each community. Within a sampled household, all persons eighteen years of age and older were rostered by proxy, and information obtained on their smoking status, thus providing estimates of community smoking prevalence. Overall, the baseline survey resulted in the identification of 162,201 eligible households with interviews completed in 88 percent of households contacted. A total of 42,170 current adult smokers were identified from the household rostering. Subsequently, telephone interviews with the rostered smokers were conducted to collect detailed information on their smoking behavior (see "endpoint cohorts" below). A second prevalence survey of smaller size will be completed at the end of the trial in 1993 to provide the data for a pre-post evaluation of change in overall community smoking prevalence.

Endpoint Cohorts

All current smokers between the ages of twenty-five and sixty-four years identified by the baseline survey roster were contacted by telephone to determine quantity and duration of cigarette smoking, other tobacco use habits, prior quit attempts, desire to quit, and demographic information. Interviews were completed with 86 percent of smokers identified from the household rostering. The baseline survey yielded approximately 500 current heavy smokers, and 1,200 light/moderate smokers in each community. From these groups, age and sex stratified cohorts of 400 heavy smokers and 400 light/moderate smokers were formed as illustrated in Figure 1. These groups were referred to as "endpoint cohorts." Both the "Light/Moderate" and "Heavy" endpoint cohorts are contacted yearly by telephone to assess smoking status. In the trial, a quitter is defined as a smoker who has not smoked for six months prior to the final follow-up interview.

Adolescent Survey

Although the COMMIT intervention is targeted to adult heavy smokers, it is possible that a community-wide campaign against smoking will also impact the smoking behavior of adolescents. For this reason, the COMMIT evaluation includes assessments of the smoking habits and attitudes of representative samples of ninth grade students in intervention and comparison communities in 1990 and 1993.

The survey of ninth grade students will be conducted by staff at each research center utilizing a standard data collection protocol and instrument. In each community, a list of ninth grade classes in public and private schools will be compiled and a random sample of classrooms will be selected to participate in the survey. A mean of eighteen ninth grade classrooms per community will be surveyed, involving approximately 450 students. Trained data collectors will administer an anonymous questionnaire in each classroom. The sample size of the youth survey has been designed to permit the detection of a 5 percent net change (from 10% to

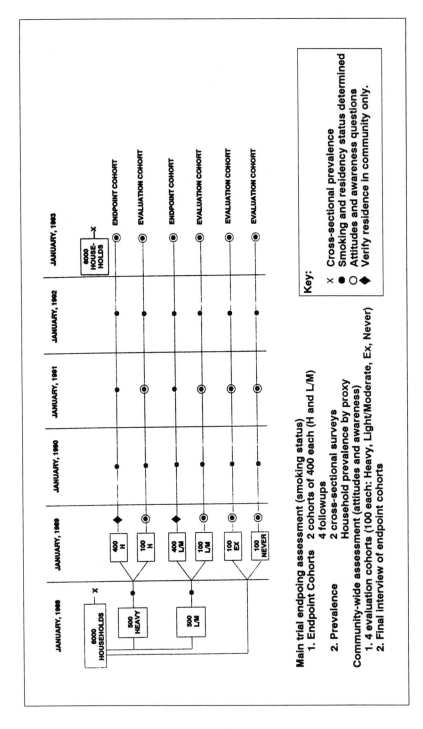

Figure 1. Surveys to assess smoking status (endpoint) and surveys to assess community-wide changes (evaluation).

15%) between intervention and comparison communities in the smoking prevalence rate among ninth graders.

IMPACT EVALUATION

The impact evaluation is designed to measure changes in factors thought to be important in facilitating community-wide smoking behavior changes. These factors include: 1) people's attitudes and beliefs about smoking and their participation in smoking control activities; 2) smoking cessation intervention practices of health care providers; 3) smoking policies and cessation programs at worksites and community organizations; 4) availability of smoking control services; and 5) the amount of media coverage given tobacco issues. The strategy for assessing each of these five factors is described below.

Assessment of the COMMIT intervention on the smoking control actions of health care providers, worksites, and organizations will be based on a posttest only comparison of survey data collected in both intervention and comparison communities in 1993. (As described below, some surveys are conducted at baseline and mid-point in intervention communities only. These data are used for intervention planning.) The decision to rely on a posttest only comparison was based on several factors. First, community analysis information and data collected in the baseline and evaluation cohort surveys indicate that community pairs are well matched and thus should not have differed greatly at baseline. Second, there was concern that the process of collecting detailed survey information at baseline from health care providers, worksites, and organizations might serve to activate these groups in the comparison communities to become more involved in smoking control activities. Finally, the posttest only design is less costly than a pre/post comparison design.

Monitoring Attitudes and Beliefs about Smoking

An important assumption underlying the COMMIT intervention is that attitudes and beliefs about smoking held by community members will be important determinants of community-wide changes in smoking behavior. To test this assumption, representative samples of smokers and nonsmokers in each community will be interviewed at three points during the trial to assess attitudes and beliefs about smoking and to determine if these changes are correlated with community-wide changes in smoking behavior.

The group of smokers and nonsmokers to be monitored for changes in knowledge, attitudes and beliefs about smoking were selected during the baseline survey. In addition to the endpoint cohorts described above, cohorts representing the population as a whole were also formed from the baseline roster in all twenty-two communities. Designated the "evaluation cohort" this group consists of 100 heavy smokers, 100 light/moderate smokers, 100 recent ex-smokers (within 5 years) and 100 nonsmokers (never smokers and long-term quitters). (See

Figure 1.) Like the endpoint cohort subjects, participants in the evaluation cohorts are contacted annually by telephone to assess smoking status. In addition, the members of the evaluation cohorts are interviewed in depth at three points during the trial (1989, 1991, and 1993), to assess the attitudinal topics summarized in Table 3. For analysis purposes, the information collected from smokers and nonsmokers will be weighted to adjust for differential sampling fractions from community populations. Additional information on community-wide attitudes and beliefs about smoking will be obtained during the 1993 final prevalence survey.

Monitoring the Smoking Cessation Practices of Health Care Providers

The COMMIT intervention includes activities intended to promote improved delivery of smoking cessation advice by health care providers [4-8]. It is hypothesized that health care providers in intervention communities will be more actively engaged in smoking control activities than health care providers in comparison communities by the end of the trial. Intervention activities aimed at health providers center around three objectives: 1) establishment of smoke-free offices; 2) regular counseling of all smokers following a standard protocol; and 3) involvement in promoting community-wide smoking control activities, e.g., the Great American Smokeout.

Two separate surveys to evaluate the impact of health provider channel will be conducted. One is a telephone survey of a sample of office practices and the other is a mailed census survey of individual practitioners. Both surveys will be performed twice during the trial in intervention communities (1990 and 1993) and once (1993) in comparison communities. The surveys are restricted to intervention communities in 1990 to avoid possible activation of comparison community health care providers. The collection of baseline information regarding the office practice characteristics and counseling practices of health care providers in intervention communities is used for intervention planning purposes, not for evaluation. Evaluation of the impact of the COMMIT intervention on health providers will be based on a posttest only comparison of survey data collected in both intervention and comparison communities in 1993.

The Health Care office survey will describe office smoking policies and cessation resources available to patients. Approximately thirty physician and thirty dental offices will be randomly selected and surveyed in each community by telephone. Eligible physicians' offices include the following primary care specialties: internal medicine, obstetrics/gynecology, osteopathy. Eligible dental offices include offices practicing general dentistry. In addition, questionnaires will be mailed to all primary care physicians and general practice dentists in each community. This survey will describe smoking cessation counseling practices of individual physicians and dentists. Major features of both surveys are summarized in Table 2. In addition to these two surveys of health care providers, data from the

Table 3. Main Topics Assessed in the Evaluation Cohort Interview

1. Current Smoking Status
   − Cigarette smoking status
   − Use of other forms of tobacco
   − Reported cessation of smoking in the past year
   − Among current smokers: amount smoked daily and type of cigarettes usually smoked (e.g., filtered vs. unfiltered; menthol vs. regular)

2. Beliefs about Cigarette Smoking
   − Dangers associated with active smoking
   − Dangers associated with passive smoke exposure
   − Among current smokers: perceived likelihood of experiencing health problems associated with smoking; perceived benefits gained by stopping smoking

3. Attitudes about Cigarette Smoking
   − Smoking as a public health problem
   − Restrictions on smoking in public places
   − Restrictions on selling tobacco to minors
   − Restrictions on advertising tobacco products

4. Social Norms Concerning Smoking
   − Usual response to smoking in public places (e.g., ask to be seated in smoking or nonsmoking section of restaurants; ask smoker not to light up around you).
   − Rules about smoking at home and in car.

5. Awareness and Participation in Smoking Control Activities
   − Awareness of: - local stop smoking programs
                         - hotline to call for help in quitting
                         - Great American Smokeout
                         - information on smoking in the media
                         - worksite smoking policies and programs

   − Participation in: - stop smoking programs
                         - hotline for cessation information
                         - Great American Smokeout
                         - worksite stop smoking programs

   − Among current smokers: - advice received from doctor and/or
                              dentist to encourage cessation

6. Demographic and Cohort Tracking Information

patient's point of view concerning physician and dentist smoking cessation counseling is collected as part of the evaluation cohort interview.

Monitoring the Smoking Control Activities of Worksites and Organizations

The COMMIT intervention includes activities intended to promote adoption of smoke-free policies, delivery of cessation services and participation in smoking control activities by worksites and community organizations. Worksites offer the opportunity to reach large numbers of smokers who may not otherwise be exposed to information about smoking. Moreover, the workplace represents a potent social environment which can help reinforce nonsmoking norms and motivate cessation attempts. Similar to worksites, community and civic organizations represent an important but underutilized channel for reaching smokers.

It is hypothesized that by the end of the trial, worksites and community organizations in intervention communities will be more likely to have adopted nonsmoking policies and to be more actively engaged in smoking control activities than worksites and organizations in comparison communities. Intervention activities aimed at worksites and community organizations center around three objectives: 1) adoption and implementation of nonsmoking policies; 2) delivery of cessation services to employees (worksites) or members (community organizations); and 3) motivation of quit attempts through incentive programs such as contests and involvement in community-wide smoking control activities.

To assess the impact of COMMIT on achievement of the intervention objectives for worksites, a representative sample of worksites with fifty or more employees will be surveyed by telephone in intervention communities in 1990 and intervention and comparison communities in 1993. The surveys will collect information about worksite characteristics (e.g., size, type of business), smoking policies, and provision of cessation services and incentives to assist employees in stopping smoking. Major features of the worksite survey are summarized in Table 2.

Worksites eligible to participate in the survey will be identified through Dun & Bradstreet listings of worksites located within the zip code/mailcode boundaries for each trial community. Dun & Bradstreet listings for each community will be supplemented by the research centers to insure a complete and up-to-date list of worksites. For the purposes of surveying and data analysis, worksites will be stratified based on number of employees, using three size strata of 50-99, 100-249, and 250 or more employees. In addition, public and private schools in each community will be surveyed as worksites.

A maximum of thirty worksites (excluding schools) per community in each of the three on-site employee size strata will be surveyed. In communities having more than thirty worksites within a given strata, thirty will be randomly selected, with replacement of refusals, to participate in the survey. In community strata having thirty or fewer worksites, all will be surveyed.

The worksite surveys will be conducted by telephone interview, carried out by a central survey contractor. The interview will be preceded by a letter sent to the company's chief executive officer (or in the case of a school, the principal) to explain the survey and to request the site to identify an appropriate contact person for the telephone interview.

In addition to the worksite survey, information concerning worksite policies, incentive programs and smoking cessation programs will be collected as part of the evaluation cohort interview.

Religious organizations will be surveyed in both intervention and comparison communities to measure the impact of the COMMIT intervention on local community organizations. Religious organizations were selected to serve as a measure of community organizations because they could be easily identified using standard criteria in all twenty-two communities and they represent an example of a community response to smoking in an elective social setting. The content of the survey instrument for religious organizations is similar to the one used for worksites.

The sampling frame for religious organizations is constructed from the yellow pages for each community. All yellow page listings under "churches" and "synagogues" within the zip code/mailcode boundaries for the community having seventy-five or more members are eligible to participate in the survey. A maximum of fifty religious organizations will be surveyed in each community. If more than fifty religious organizations exist, a random sample of fifty will be selected with replacement of refusals.

The survey of religious organizations will be carried at the same time and will use the same interview methodology as the worksite survey. Major features of the survey of religious organizations are summarized in Table 2.

Monitoring Community Smoking Control Services

The COMMIT intervention is intended to stimulate community organizations to expand their offerings of cessation assistance and information to the public. It is hypothesized that the availability and utilization of smoking control services will be increased to a greater extent in intervention communities compared to comparison communities.

Cessation Resource Surveys to monitor changes in the availability and utilization of smoking control services will be carried out in both intervention and comparison communities at baseline (Fall 1989), at the midpoint of the trial (Fall 1991), and at the end of the intervention (Fall 1993). The intent of the surveys is to establish a baseline level of the availability and utilization of smoking control services in intervention and control communities and then to track changes in these services over the course of the trial.

The sampling frame for cessation resource surveys consists of seven categories of organizations: 1) voluntary agencies (i.e., American Lung Association, American Cancer Society, etc.); 2) hospitals; 3) city and county medical and dental societies; 4) health maintenance organizations; 5) county or regional medical and dental societies; 6) public libraries; and 7) proprietary smoking cessation programs. In each community, organizations will be identified by examining local white and yellow page directories and indexed sections of Polk/ Henderson type directories. All eligible organizations will be contacted to participate in the survey.

The surveys will be administered over the telephone by staff at each research center following a standard protocol. A letter will be sent to organizations in advance of the telephone interview to explain the survey and to request organizations to identify appropriate people to be interviewed. Each organization contacted is asked to provide information on provision of a variety of smoking control services including: stop smoking classes, distribution of stop smoking guides and educational materials, sponsorship of anti-smoking events, and sponsorship of worksite and health provider workshops. For each service offered, the organization will be asked to report the frequency that the service is offered and the level of community participation (e.g., attendance at stop smoking classes). Major features of the cessation resource surveys are summarized in Table 2.

In addition to the cessation resource surveys, data concerning utilization of smoking cessation aids and participation in smoking related activities are collected as part of the evaluation cohort interview of current smokers.

Media Tracking

The COMMIT intervention includes activities intended to increase local coverage of tobacco issues by broadcast and print media. The effective use of the mass media to promote nonsmoking norms and actions is viewed as critical to the trial's success in reducing the prevalence of smoking. COMMIT activities directed at media coverage of tobacco issues fall into four categories: 1) awareness designed to educate the public about smoking; 2) community-wide magnet events designed to promote smoking cessation (e.g., Great American Smokeout, Quit and Win contests); 3) promotion of local cessation services (e.g., stop smoking hotline); and 4) media advocacy to increase news coverage of smoking control issues and public recognition of smoking as a public health problem. It is hypothesized that media coverage of tobacco issues will increase over the course of the trial and will be greater in intervention communities compared to comparison communities.

Media coverage of tobacco issues is monitored by a commercial clipping service that scans local and regional newspapers serving each of the twenty-two COMMIT communities for articles and ads on tobacco. Every newspaper clip is coded following a standard protocol according to the following: 1) format (i.e., ad, announcement, hard news, feature, editorial, letter to the editor, obituary, cartoon); 2) length (i.e., column inches); 3) focus (i.e., pro or anti-tobacco); 4) message feature (i.e., information, motivation, instruction, modeling); 5) keyword used to identify the clip; and 6) newspaper. Newspaper clipping began in the Fall of 1988 and will continue until January 1993. The primary indicator of change in media coverage of tobacco issues will be based on the change in total column inches devoted to anti-tobacco coverage between baseline (October-December 1988) and the end of the trial (October-December 1993) between intervention and comparison communities. Local broadcast media are not being monitored, due to the high cost of establishing such a surveillance system. Monitoring newspapers is felt to provide a reasonable proxy measure of tobacco coverage by broadcast media.

A cohort of twenty billboards located in high traffic areas of each community is being monitored bi-annually to assess changes in the prevalence of pro- and anti-tobacco advertisements. One community, Santa Fe, New Mexico, has a local ordinance prohibiting billboards and will not be monitored. In addition to monitoring newspaper clips and billboards, information on the public's awareness of tobacco news and events in the media is also collected as part of the evaluation cohort interview.

PROCESS EVALUATION

Process evaluation is designed to document the performance of the intervention activities to and provide information to aid interpretation of outcome and impact results. COMMIT process evaluation includes three components: 1) a computerized program records system containing information on the performance of mandated intervention activities in intervention communities; 2) quarterly reports from the research center staff which provide a means for gathering interpretative descriptions of intervention activities and the community mobilization process; and 3) a community tracking system which provides a way to record information about the unique characteristics of intervention and comparison communities which may be important in interpreting results (e.g., legislative changes, important community issues). These three components of the process evaluation plan are described below, and in more detail by Corbett et al. [10].

Program Records System

The COMMIT intervention protocol includes fifty-one required activities. In an effort to standardize the COMMIT intervention across communities, a timetable and minimum performance standards were specified for each required activity. The program records system was established as a standardized way to document the extent to which required intervention activities are performed. The system is the mechanism by which the trial monitors each site's progress in completing mandated activities, and which will ultimately provide a quantitative measure of the "dose" of intervention delivered in each community.

COMMIT field staff record information on activity performance using standard program record forms. Information collected on these forms includes: type of activity, date of performance, number of participants, cost of the activity, and staff and volunteer time devoted to the activity. Hardcopy program record forms are continually computerized using a customized software program developed for COMMIT. The computerized records system is used to generate summary indicators of activity performance and to compare activity performance across sites. Independent program record audits are performed periodically by NCI staff to validate information entered into the program records system and monitor quality of protocol implementation.

Quarterly Reports

Each research center produces a standardized written report summarizing project activities at the end of each quarter. The Quarterly Reports include descriptions of activities in four areas: 1) health care providers; 2) worksites and organizations; 3) public education; and 4) cessation resources and services. In addition, the reports contain information on community board and task force activities. Twice a year each research site prepares case history reports which provide detailed information on performance of selected activities. Field staff and researchers at each site collaborate to produce the report.

The Quarterly Report serves multiple functions. It provides another means for the trial to monitor site differences in intervention performance. It also serves as a way for research centers to share information about intervention activities. Finally, it is hoped that at the end of the trial the reports will be helpful in understanding outcome and impact results. The information presented in the Quarterly Reports should facilitate dissemination of trial results to other settings. Since the reports provide descriptions of activity performance, problems pertaining to implementation of activities will be known and can be taken into account in planning for dissemination.

Community Tracking

Community tracking includes the monitoring of events, legislation, and programs in communities which may affect smoking patterns but which may not be directly related to COMMIT; for example, local ordinances regulating smoking in public places. Documenting these secular changes occurring in both intervention and comparison communities is necessary to understand the trial results.

Community tracking for COMMIT includes the following: 1) biannual documentation of local and state laws regulating tobacco; 2) monitoring local daily newspapers to identify important community events and issues; and 3) periodically interviewing key informants to identify important community issues relevant to tobacco use (e.g., formation of a coalition to address youth access to tobacco). Legislative tracking information will be collected using a standard form and entered into the program records system. Summaries derived from monitoring newspaper coverage of community events and issues and key informant interviews are included in the Quarterly Reports prepared by each research center.

ECONOMIC EVALUATION

Ultimately, it is the goal of the COMMIT evaluation to yield information that will guide future efforts to reduce tobacco use in an efficient and economical way. As a part of the trial's evaluation, an economic analysis will estimate the marginal societal cost of increased levels of smoking cessation obtained via the COMMIT intervention. The focus on marginal societal costs rather than programmatic costs is based on the assumption that it is unlikely that the level of COMMIT program expenditures will be replicated in the future. Thus, the economic analysis will be directed at estimating the benefit that would be expected to be derived at different levels of investment in COMMIT-type activities.

Another important aspect of the economic analysis is estimation of the extent to which the COMMIT intervention helped stimulate increases in the allocation of community resources to smoking cessation activities. The concept that COMMIT will induce an overall increase in community smoking control activities is central to the community-based intervention approach. The economic analysis integrates all three levels of evaluation plan (i.e., outcome, impact, and process assessment) in an effort to provide information that will be useful to policy makers in helping them make decisions about how and where to allocate scarce societal resources.

CONCLUSIONS

The COMMIT evaluation is designed to monitor changes in community smoking patterns and to allow testing of the assumptions which have guided the development of the intervention.

The nature of the COMMIT intervention and study design will not permit a direct assessment of the effect of specific intervention activities on smoking behavior. Rather, the evaluation will allow for the measurement of the aggregate effect of a community wide intervention with many facets. The evaluation plan reflects the underlying assumption that reductions in community smoking behavior are best accomplished through the combined effects of intervention activities implemented simultaneously through multiple community channels.

ACKNOWLEDGMENTS

The authors thank Norman Hymowitz, Russell Glasgow, Charles Goldsmith, Russell Sciandra, and the members of the COMMIT Design and Evaluation Committee for their helpful comments on earlier drafts.

REFERENCES

1. P. Greenwald and E. Sondik, Cancer Control Objectives for the Nation: 1985-2000, *NCI Monographs, 2*, pp. 3-74, 1986.
2. U.S. Department of Health and Human Services, *The Health Consequences of Smoking: Cancer. A Report of the Surgeon General*, U.S. Department of Health and Human Services, Public Health Service, Office on Smoking and Health, DHHS Publication No. (PHS) 82-50179, 1982.
3. COMMIT Research Group, *The Community Intervention Trial for Smoking Cessation: Protocol Summary*, National Cancer Institute, 1988.
4. L. Wallack and R. Sciandra, Media Advocacy and Public Education in the Community Intervention Trial to Reduce Heavy Smoking (COMMIT), *International Quarterly of Community Health Education, 11*:3, pp. 205-222, 1990-91.
5. J. K. Ockene, E. L. Lindsay, L. Berger, and N. Hymowitz, Health Care Providers as Key Change Agents in the Community Intervention Trial for Smoking Cessation (COMMIT), *International Quarterly of Community Health Education, 11*:3, pp. 223-237, 1990-91
6. G. Sorensen, R. E. Glasgow, and K. Corbett, Promoting Smoking Control through Worksites in the Community Intervention Trial for Smoking Cessation (COMMIT), *International Quarterly of Community Health Education, 11*:3, pp. 239-257, 1990-91.
7. B. Thompson, L. Wallack, E. Lichtenstein, and T. Pechacek, Principles of Community Organization and Partnership for Smoking Cessation in the Community Intervention Trial for Smoking Cessation (COMMIT), *International Quarterly of Community Health Education, 11*:3, pp. 187-203, 1990-91.
8. P. Pomrehn, R. Sciandra, R. Shipley, W. Lynn, and H. Lando, Enhancing Resources for Smoking Cessation through Community Intervention: COMMIT as a Prototype, *International Quarterly of Community Health Education, 11*:3, pp. 259-269, 1990-91.
9. D. Byar, M. Gail, M. Green, D. Corle, and T. F. Pechacek, Statistical Design of the Community Intervention Trial for Smoking Cessation, ms submitted for publication.
10. K. Corbett, B. Thompson, N. White, and M. Taylor, Process Evaluation in the Community Intervention Trial for Smoking Cessation (COMMIT), *International Quarterly of Community Health Education, 11*:3, pp. 291-309, 1990-91.

Direct reprint requests to:

Margaret E. Mattson, Ph.D.
National Institute on Alcohol Abuse and Alcholism
Parklawn Building, Rm 14C-20
5600 Fishers Lane
Rockville, MD 20857

PROCESS EVALUATION IN THE COMMUNITY INTERVENTION TRIAL FOR SMOKING CESSATION (COMMIT)

KITTY CORBETT
Kaiser Permanente Medical Care Programs
Oakland, CA

BETI THOMPSON
Fred Hutchinson Cancer Research Center
Seattle, Washington

NORMAN WHITE

MARTIN TAYLOR

McMaster University
Hamilton, Ontario

For the COMMIT Research Group

ABSTRACT

The reach and complexity of the multi-site Community Intervention Trial for Smoking Cessation (COMMIT) project call for an extensive, comprehensive evaluation plan. This article reports on the objectives, methods, and data sets of the part of the plan designed for process evaluation. We describe the systems developed for: monitoring progress in the sites, the quality of local intervention activities and data collection, and compliance with the trial-wide protocol; disseminating information for formative purposes; and generating and using process data for outcome evaluation. The process evaluation approach includes both quantitative and qualitative methods. We provide examples from community mobilization and intervention in different communities.

Int'l. Quarterly of Community Health Education, Vol. 11(3) 291-309, 1990-91

© 1991, Baywood Publishing Co., Inc.

The Community Intervention Trial for Smoking Cessation (COMMIT) is a National Cancer Institute study of a strategy to increase cessation rates among heavy smokers in eleven North American locales. The COMMIT intervention is a package of fifty-one mandated activities codified in the official project protocol [1-5]. The protocol gives minimum impact objectives and process objectives for each activity, and sets minimum criteria for standardization of the interventions across sites. Specifics of local implementation, however, are determined by community boards and task forces as described elsewhere in this issue [5].

The project's reach and complexity present a challenge for process evaluation. Process evaluation needs include: assessing the impact of mediating factors (e.g., social norms; media messages supporting nonsmoking; the impact of legislation) postulated to lead to changes in smoking rates; and monitoring community mobilization and delivery of the interventions. A comprehensive process evaluation plan has been devised to address those research needs. The plan includes two main components: 1) a monitoring structure for the assessment of compliance with the protocol and quality control of both activities and data, and sharing of trial activities among the eleven intervention sites; and 2) a structure for providing information for summative needs, including the assessment of the relationship of project activities to outcomes, and the identification and examination of competing explanations for findings at the end of the trial.

This article describes the system in COMMIT for monitoring and evaluating progress in the intervention and, to lesser extent, comparison communities. It addresses the ways COMMIT is tracking the community mobilization process, assessing the implementation of intervention activities, and identifying the existence of competing community events and issues which might provide alternative explanations for findings. It describes an innovative methodology which uses both qualitative and quantitative methods in process evaluation, and provides examples of the monitoring system from the first year of community mobilization and intervention. The COMMIT experiment involves both a set of prescribed interventions and the community-based organization for their delivery. The project provides an unprecedented opportunity to evaluate not only the effects of this state-of-the-art approach to smoking cessation, but also the processes through which community boards, task forces, and staff implement a protocol in diverse sites.

DATA FOR PROCESS EVALUATION IN COMMIT

The literature on the evaluation of social programs stresses that a key challenge in process evaluation is the matching of methods to objectives and audiences [6-10]. Evaluations use systematic methods to assess whether programs have met their objectives, how program activities were implemented, what other factors might explain outcomes, and whether the programs are useful. At a minimum, evaluations address outcomes and processes. Evaluators employ differing definitions of terms to describe outcomes and processes.

Outcome evaluation may or may not be synonymous with "impact evaluation," and serves the role of "summative evaluation" to assess the effectiveness of a program in meeting its impact objectives and overall goals for change. Program outcome or impact evaluations usually rely on comparison of baseline data collected on individuals prior to the program with data collected after the program's conclusion, and must ultimately take into account non-program influences on outcomes.

Process evaluation addresses what the intervention program consists of, how activities serve short-term objectives, how activities are carried out, and what other factors contribute to outcomes. It may entail "implementation evaluation," "quality control," "quality assurance review," "program utility assessment," "process analysis," and other assessments. Process evaluation can have a "formative" role during the development and unfolding of a program as well as a "summative" function. Quantitative process objectives along a timeline are often employed to facilitate evaluation of program delivery. Process evaluation may be designed to provide information to feed back suggestions to program designers, for mid-course corrections. For some researchers, process evaluation may also refer to qualitative assessment of the dynamics of program operations [10]. Ultimately, what is needed is to know what specific results were and how they came about.

In a project with the scope of COMMIT, process evaluation serves many ends. To ensure maximum return from the trial, it is crucial that at the project's conclusion data exist which allow the generation of explanatory constructs. The data must satisfy certain criteria. They must be collected about relevant structures, events, and processes. They must be constructed competently, in standardized fashion. They must be summarized, stored, interpreted, and disseminated in ways which permit site-specific, inter-site, and trial-wide inferences. These requirements have led to the development of an assortment of instruments and codified procedures, e.g., uniform rules for record-keeping, training for research staff, detailed manuals of operation, a system for regular electronic communication among sites, and effective data management.

Data for evaluating the trial are being collected through various means. Centrally conducted surveys are generating the baseline, interim, and endpoint counts with which to test the fundamental smoking outcome questions. To assess attainment of impact and process objectives, COMMIT has over a dozen evaluation surveys and tracking protocols. The rationale and methodology of the overall evaluation plan, with special attention to the determination of changes in smoking behavior, are discussed elsewhere [11].

Beyond survey data, an assortment of data constitutes the "Project Archives" for COMMIT. They form a compendium of materials about the communities and COMMIT activities. These data sources include textual profiles of

Table 1. Data Elements in the Project Archives

| | Community | | |
	Intervention	Comparison	Frequency
Community Analysis	x	x	baseline
Program Records	x		6/year
Quarterly Reports Forms			quarterly
Overview/Highlights	x		quarterly
Contextual tracking, e.g., legislation	x	x	quarterly
Community mobilization	x		quarterly
Task force activities	x		
Public education	x		quarterly
Health care	x		quarterly
Worksites/Organizations	x		quarterly
Cessation resources	x		quarterly
Local newspapers; major issues	x	x	quarterly
Case histories	x		quarterly
Minutes and handouts	x		ongoing
Local correspondence	x		ongoing
Media			
Billboard tracking	x	x	2/yr
Newspaper clippings	x	x	ongoing
Information on tobacco industry actions	x	x	ongoing

the communities, spreadsheets on expenditures of money and time, records for tracking program, media, and legislative activities in each community, narrative reports on mobilization and intervention, and other local materials (e.g., minutes from meetings, correspondence). The Project Archives are designed to complement the various process and outcome surveys, provide an integrated framework for evaluation and trial management, and provide an interpretive context for both process and outcome evaluation. The system allows for the ongoing generation and collation of a variety of qualitative and quantitative data, together with local interpretation of them, which are regularly reduced and can be juxtaposed against available survey findings.

The Project Archives, as shown in Table 1, include data from a wide variety of sources. Components of the archives which are of special interest for process evaluation are discussed later. The data vary from counts, such as the number of newspaper articles devoted to smoking events and issues, to interpretations of community activities, such as case histories of specific smoking control efforts. The components of the Archives serve different purposes: for example, the Program Records System is most useful for tracking the intervention activities in the intervention communities; the Media Tracking System assesses media attention to the smoking issue in both intervention and comparison communities; and the Quarterly Reports provide interpretive accounts of smoking-related and nonsmoking-related events and activities in both comparison and intervention communities.

Smoking-related events and trends are being monitored in the comparison communities, but information about them is collected primarily through the centrally conducted evaluation surveys [11]. Some of the process evaluation data being collected for intervention sites, such as reports of community mobilization and activities for smoking and tobacco control, is only minimally collected for comparison sites. This is to avoid the possibility that the queries and presence of researchers might stimulate greater smoking control activity in those communities, and thereby influence results. Early in the project, community analyses of the comparison communities as well as intervention communities were carried out, to identify baseline differences between pairs of communities. Throughout the trial, the comparison sites are monitored for changes, events, and activities that may affect smoking or smoking cessation rates. Primary sources of information within the comparison community include reading and coding of daily newspapers, interviews with key informants, use of available secondary data, and unobtrusive observation of selected smoking control events. All of the above data gathering activities are constrained by protocol guidelines designed to minimize visibility of the trial in the comparison communities.

The bulk of process data is being collected in the intervention communities. Although it is premature to assess the overall relevance of the process variables to trial outcomes, the Project Archives data have already been useful in monitoring the mobilization process, as well as early intervention activities [5, 12]. The specific pieces of the Project Archives that have been most important for monitoring purposes are described below.

Community Analysis Documents

Prior to randomization of the eleven matched pairs of communities into intervention and comparison sites, review of secondary sources and interviews with key informants were used to produce a "community profile" of all twenty-two COMMIT communities. Following randomization, further investigation in the intervention communities led to the production of "Community Analysis" documents, which were reviewed, modified, and validated by community board representatives. In addition to describing resources, sectors of influence, leaders, and the history of collaborative and public health efforts in the community, force field analysis delineated facilitating and inhibiting factors in the community that might affect COMMIT [13, 14]. The qualitative, baseline descriptions in the Community Analyses are useful for assessing features of the community context which are of potential importance to mobilization activities and achievement of objectives. In light of variation among the sites in relevant background experiences (e.g., a history of volunteerism, community health promotion projects, and smoking control efforts such as lobbying for a local smoking ordinance), such constructs include the experience and readiness of a community to initiate COMMIT activities [5].

Program Records

The term "Program Records" refers to quantitative data in a versatile and comprehensive computerized relational data base. The system serves multiple trial functions, such as the documentation of COMMIT activities and the participation of local individuals and organizations. It was designed to meet the need for an efficient system to capture, retrieve, display, and report information over the course of the study.

Field staff fill out standardized forms and then use the Program Records software system to key-in information about affiliates (people and organizations in the community involved with COMMIT), presentations, consultations, events, media activity, distributed materials, and time spent by staff and volunteers on activities. The program records whether and when mandated activities occurred, if the process objectives were achieved, and details about the specific activities. Summary reports tally findings from all sites. Local reports can also be generated on the affiliates, activities, media messages, and other details about different activities.

This data base is the principal means by which central COMMIT staff and Steering Committee members ascertain the status of different sites with respect to mandated activities, and the status of the activities across all sites. Bi-monthly submission of data from each site is required.

Quarterly Reports

The Quarterly Reports are both descriptive and interpretive. They contain both written narratives and answers to standardized checklists. Field staff and researchers at each site collaborate to address several sets of questions. The responses provide:

- an overview and highlights of activities
- a summary of contextual changes, including local activities of tobacco industry activities

- tracking of local and state legislation pertinent to tobacco issues
- monitoring of daily newspapers for events and programs in the community which may affect smoking patterns, COMMIT developments and outcomes
- an update on community mobilization activities
- summaries of activities for the four task force areas
  - Health Care Providers
  - Worksites and Organizations
  - Public Education
  - Cessation Resources and Services
- case history reports on selected activities

Attachments to each Quarterly Report include minutes from board and task force meetings, handouts, and printed materials produced by each site.

The Quarterly Reports follow the intervention as it is implemented in the different sites and are another means of ensuring the integrity of the trial. This package is useful to identify innovations which might be diffused elsewhere, and to detect problems so that appropriate and prompt mid-course corrections can be made. It thus serves both quality control and formative evaluation needs. It may also serve a summative evaluation function, in providing information for interpreting outcome and impact findings. Regular reviews of the Quarterly Reports facilitate the definition and tracking of variables that may explain differences between sites in achieving trial goals and objectives.

A number of variables have been detected as potential mediating forces on trial outcomes, and suggest rival hypotheses for the explanation of findings at the end of the trial. For example, an increase in tobacco industry activities in the intervention communities may influence the outcome of the trial. Additionally, state legislative initiatives, such as the passage in California of Proposition 99 (whose additional tax on cigarette is funding a massive statewide education, intervention, and research campaign), may lead to widespread reductions in smoking prevalence which could overwhelm our ability to find a difference between a pair of COMMIT communities. On a more prosaic level, in the intervention communities, tensions between the individuals and groups that administer the local project may slow down the implementation of the intervention, reducing the likelihood of achieving the trial goals. The data source for this type of information is the Quarterly Reports. In comparison sites, data from the surveys, tracking of newspapers, and interviews with select key informants will provide information to evaluate other rival hypotheses, such as the diffusion of treatment from an intervention site to its matched pair, compensatory rivalry or stepped-up activities in the comparison site as a response to being in the study, or other aspects of local history which could affect results.

USE OF THE PROJECT ARCHIVES
FOR MONITORING PROGRESS

Information from the Project Archives has several major functions in process evaluation of the trial in the intervention sites. These include: monitoring of compliance with the specifications of the protocol; culling of information for dissemination to all sites, including the identification of valuable ideas and innovations; and the recognition of potential problems (e.g., in adherence to requirements for record-keeping and the delivery of interventions) which require attention.

Compliance with the Protocol

A trial of the magnitude of COMMIT requires regular monitoring to be certain that the integrity of the trial is maintained as project objectives are met. Quality control review monitors whether sites are implementing mandated activities as specified by criteria in the protocol, and in a manner which reflects the "spirit" of the protocol (i.e., that much authority rests with members of the local community boards and task forces). The unfolding developments in the communities are monitored to keep tabs on similarities and differences in the delivery of interventions in the relevant sites; it documents that at least the minimum "dose" is provided to all sites in the COMMIT experiment. It is essential to know that sites are delivering the package as mandated, so that the study hypothesis can be validly tested. Deviation from the protocol would make it difficult to attribute results to the intervention.

The quality of delivery of interventions, the quantity of activities conducted, and the degree to which process objectives are achieved are being assessed through a *quality control review*. Quality control audits by a central Quality Control Committee include the evaluation of sites' progress through review of Quarterly Reports, data from Program Records, and the construction of summary scores (constructed using data from the Program Records system). The quality control system serves to assess the quality of activities carried out as well as of the data collected.

The quality control review involves two phases. In the first phase, all data records about intervention activities and attainment of process objectives are reviewed by a Quality Control Committee made up of study investigators. Activities which have incomplete information, are questionable in terms of the protocol, or are judged to be inconsistent with the protocol, are flagged. Reviewers check the primary data files from the site in question, and discuss the matter with field staff. After discussion, a determination is made about whether an activity "qualifies" or not for meeting a process objective. Action on recommended changes is checked at later submissions of Program Records data.

In the second phase of the audit, a 10 percent random sample of activities per site is selected. Field sites where the activity occurred are telephoned and asked to

Table 2. Site-Specific Implementation of Mandated Activity:
Comprehensive Training of Physicians

Due Date: 9/30/89

*Process Objective: 10% of primary care physicians in the community
will have received comprehensive training*

Site	Date[a]	Training Length (Hours)	Number of Targeted Physicians Attending/ Total MDs[b]	Percent Process Objective Attained	Media Coverage?
A	11/21	1.0	20/87	0	No
B	9/14	3.0	6/82	70	No
C	4/19 & 7/30	2.5	7/70	100	No
D	9/27	6.0	8/132	60	No
E	none	NA	0/88	0	NA
F	11/13	3.0	4/114	40	Yes
G	9/28	3.3	7/81	90	No
H	10/05	3.0	21/167	125	No
I	10/18	4.0	9/78	115	No
J	9/23	3.5	5/98	50	No
K	10/28	6.0	14/59	240	Yes

Note: NA = Not Applicable.
[a] The date notation used here is month/day.
[b] Estimated number of physicians in the community.

describe details about what took place. Hard copies of the relevant data collection forms are mailed immediately after the conversation. If all are consistent with the protocol, no further action is taken. Otherwise, adjustments are recommended. Any sites which have repeated problems are subject to a more extensive review, which may include a visit to the site for problem-solving.

Tables 2 and 3 illustrate progress in two protocol-mandated activities as assessed from data in the Program Records system. They are reports on the status of the sites with respect to attainment of specific process objectives, in the case of the activity "Comprehensive Training of Physicians" in Table 2, and "Annual Smoking Policy Workshop" for large worksites in Table 3. In the first of these activities, physicians receive at least two-and-one-half hours of training about smoking and how to counsel patients in smoking cessation. By the end of November 1989, ten of the eleven sites had conducted at least one comprehensive training, although several

Table 3. Site-Specific Implementation of Mandated Activity:
Annual Smoking Policy Workshop for Large Worksites

Due Date: 9/30/89

Process Objective: Conduct one workshop

Site	Date[a]	Number of Targeted Worksites Attending/Total Worksites[b]	Percent Targeted Worksites Attending	Media Coverage?
A	11/13	4/45	9	No
B	9/12	7/77	9	Yes
C	9/26	13/67	19	Yes
D	9/18 & 11/8	17/176	28	No
E	11/17	4/55	20	Yes
F	9/19	17/112	15	Yes
G	9/18	18/85	21	No
H	11/14	24/274	9	Yes
I	none	0/79	0	NA
J	9/27	12/66	18	Yes
K	6/20	12/44	27	Yes

Note: NA = Not Applicable.
[a] The date notation used here is month/day.
[b] Estimated number of targeted worksites in the community.

were unable to meet the criteria for satisfying the specific process objective. In Santa Fe, New Mexico, a training was scheduled but canceled due to lack of interest. Sites differed in their ability to attract physicians to the training. In other sites, attendance was low or the duration of the training was less than mandated. The long-term goal, providing comprehensive training to 25 percent of all primary care physicians, was met in one site, Bellingham, Washington. The table also draws on other information available in Program Records–documentation of media coverage–which may lead to sharing of ideas and problem-solving to increase participation. These data illustrate compliance with minimum criteria, but are not expressive of the variation in how activities were carried out across sites.

The comment files in Program Records add some detail about how activities occurred. In the same example described above, some sites had a two-and-one-half hour session with local physicians which offered training. Other sites had a session that lasted an entire day, offered the session in conjunction with training for office staff, and involved nationally-known speakers as trainers. While not part of the quality control plan, such details are valuable for the dissemination of information (described below).

Table 3 indicates that by the end of November 1989, all but one site had met the protocol requirement for conducting a two to three hour smoking policy workshop for representatives of worksites. For this activity, targeted large worksites are defined as those with more than 100 employees, at least 30 percent of whom reside in the community. Although there was no numerical target expressed in a process objective for the first year, good progress was made in many sites towards meeting later targets. Although some sites, such as Brantford, Ontario, experienced repeated setbacks by turn-over in task force composition and leadership, in general, the workshops were well attended.

Summary scores are constructed periodically for each site, in response to a request from COMMIT's Policy Advisory Committee for a succinct, quantitative, representation or trialwide "snapshot" assessment of overall progress by sites. Given the dozens of activities required for each site in COMMIT, as well as the great variety of process objectives considered necessary for a significant impact on smoking rates, the summary score is a concise and efficient, albeit highly reduced, measure.

The summary scores include quantitative and qualitative dimensions. A count of mandated activities that have been initiated and completed is adjusted for the degree to which process objectives have been achieved for the activities. Since other factors which are not captured in the score can influence progress (e.g., local organizational strategies for the early mobilization phase, competing events in the community, challenges in recruitment of a targeted audience, turnover in board and task force membership, etc.), the score cannot be regarded as a complete assessment of site-specific performance. Although from a management as well as analytic perspective, the summary score lacks completeness, its utility lies in providing an overview of trialwide as well as site-specific progress.

Methods for computing a summary score are somewhat arbitrary, and a decision was made to seek a compromise between merely conducting an activity and achieving its process objectives. It was deemed inappropriate to "count" an activity that, although carried out, failed to reach any part of the process objective established for it. Similarly, given the enormous amount of mobilization required in the first year of intervention, it was not considered appropriate to require attainment of 100 percent of the process objective for a particular activity to "count." The compromise measure, illustrated in Table 4, is a summary measure that gives a site credit for conducting an activity and attaining at least 75 percent of the process objective. As can be seen from that table, sites were progressing well in attaining objectives.

Table 4. Summary Scores: At Least 75 Percent of Process Objectives Attained

Channel	Intervention Communities											
	A	B	C	D	E	F	G	H	I	J	K	Average
Mobilization of Community Planning Group	100	100	100	100	89	100	100	100	100	100	100	99
Mobilization of Task Forces	100	100	100	100	100	100	89	100	89	100	100	98
Health Care Providers Task Force Area	88	83	38	50	38	75	30	83	88	75	75	54
Worksites and Organizations Task Force	55	44	87	39	44	44	55	89	87	87	78	64
Cessation Resources and Services Task Force	50	100	100	50	100	0	50	50	100	100	100	73
Public Education Task Force Area	90	80	70	80	30	90	40	90	100	70	90	78
TOTAL SCORE: (for 47 Process Objectives)	85	79	77	85	86	79	88	87	89	83	89	81

Information Dissemination

There are many mechanisms built into the trial to facilitate information sharing, including an elaborate electronic mail system, regular meetings of the various groups involved in the project, and distribution of project materials to all sites. One of the functions of the Quarterly Reports is to contribute to the overall information flow.

The volume of information available from eleven sites is massive. Identification of information from single sites which is useful for others is a challenge; so is its reduction and packaging. Three forms in the Quarterly Reports address this need. They provide summary information about overall progress, the status of mobilization, and task force activities. Copies of these forms are shared across all sites. Through the first year of mobilization and early months of the intervention phase, reports were prepared which summarized progress overall, described how sites carried out various activities, and reported on frustrations and "amazing facts" that might be of interest to other sites. The Quarterly Reports are reviewed then both by all sites and by the project's coordinating center for identification of problem areas that need to be examined on a trial-wide basis.

An important purpose for the system of sharing information is the identification of innovative activities and "good ideas." Just as there is a synergy between activities within a community, there can also be a synergy between communities as original or resourceful activities and plans are shared. Innovative and unusual activities, and reports of dealing with unexpected obstacles and possibilities, are described in the summary forms of the Quarterly Reports. The New Mexico site, for example, has had success with publicity that uses the motif of a coyote; some other sites have been stimulated to develop their own visual "mascots." Different sites have developed gimmicks for attracting smokers to sign up on the network; these ideas are shared and in turn generate new ideas. Examples include the layout of a "network card," colorful posters and banners, and the use of body-size cigarette and turkey costumes to attract attention in parades. Most promising to date are ideas for competitions and prizes: "Quit and Win" contests, for instance, held community wide or in worksites. Other useful shared ideas are related to the myriad and non-trivial tasks of COMMIT record-keeping and administration.

The Quarterly Reports both document and foster innovations in other sites. These texts thus serve as a stimulus for creativity by highlighting a wide range of strategies and options possible in carrying out COMMIT mandates.

Detection of Potential Problems

A final function of the Project Archives system is to provide a mechanism for detection of potential problems, so that timely solutions can be found. Problems to date include some having to do simply with monitoring and record keeping, thereby serving as feedback in the loop refining that system. Other problems relate to the mobilization process and the implementation of the

COMMIT interventions. An ongoing issue is the interpretation of whether a task force activity, as proposed and carried out in a site, satisfies the criteria for meeting a specific process objective.

Both Program Records and the Quarterly Reports serve this troubleshooting need. Reports from the Program Records system indicate at a glance which objectives have been met satisfactorily and which remain to be done. Other data sources are also useful for turning up existing or potential problems. In the forms in the Quarterly Reports, a checklist of information on mobilization activities lists the number of meetings of the board, task forces, and subcommittees, plus attendance at each, expressed in raw numbers and in percentages of total membership of the particular committee. Chronically low attendance at meetings, or rarity of scheduled meetings, may signal to the trialwide quality control committee, as well as local staff, a problem at the site.

Textual descriptions in the Quarterly Reports are another means of identifying potential problems, whether site-specific or trialwide. When virtually every site reported frustration with the timeline and the procedures for setting up a field office, requirements were modified trial-wide. When a site reports disagreements between the community board and the research institution on management issues, these can be assessed in light of the protocol and experiences at other sites, and suggestions can be made for revised procedures or policies. If a task force disagrees with the protocol about the value of a mandated COMMIT activity, the opinion and related activity, or inactivity in this case, are reported in the Quarterly Report. Within the reports, case histories and interviews with key informants about the changing culture of smoking also lend themselves to assessing the appropriateness of the activities and media messages employed in the community. When process evaluation indicates a need, mid-course modifications are possible.

USES OF THE MONITORING DATA
FOR OUTCOME EVALUATION

Variables and constructs developed from the Project Archives data for project management and process evaluation will also serve COMMIT's needs in outcome evaluation, to supplement information from the project's evaluation surveys (described elsewhere) [11]. Within the Project Archives, the Program Records system contains details on "what" happens in the sites as activities are carried out. Descriptive and interpretive data, as produced for the Quarterly Reports, are more appropriate for addressing "why" and "how" questions about the process [10, 15, 16]. Beyond identifying a trial effect, evaluation efforts will draw on data in the Project Archives to answer the following questions:

1. *What actually happened in the sites*: What exactly was implemented? Were there substantial differences in the ways activities were implemented in the eleven sites?

2. *How it happened*: What was the process by which community people came to the project, "bought into" the COMMIT concept, carried out the activities, and resolved problems that came up?
3. *What else happened*: What else was going on which might provide competing explanations for our outcomes?

The Quarterly Reports and the other pieces of archival material in the project fill out the accounts of the computerized data bank with narrative interpretations, and monitor other aspects of the communities.

Descriptions and interpretation of events and trends are sensibly approached at two levels: within and across communities. The raw data in the Project Archives pertain to individual sites. Each community represents a case study in itself and, despite the parallels with ten other sites following the same protocol, can be examined for its own individual history of mobilization and intervention activities. At this level, critical events, such as strong support, or resistance, by community leaders, or passage of a smoking control ordinance, may emerge in a specific site that directly affect the course of the trial, the completion of activities, and the achievement of objectives. At least two intervention sites, for example, have witnessed attempts to form "Smokers' Rights" groups in their communities. Those communities may encounter more resistance in meeting project goals than others which have no organized opposition groups. Other sites have already passed local ordinances eliminating smoking in public buildings. In those communities, it may be easier to meet project goals regarding control of smoking in public places. Each community will be examined individually so that such events can be described and assessed.

The second level of description and interpretation is the examination of commonalities in experience across sites. Sites will be grouped based on outcome measures (e.g., high, average, and low increase in cessation rates) and both similar and contrasting events and trends within and between groups will be identified. The ability to detect effects and the associated strength of inference will vary with the specificity of the relationships involved.

The data gathered will be used to understand the relationship of outcome differences across sites to 1) protocol adherence and 2) mobilization and other process factors.

The Relationship of Outcome Differences Across Sites to Protocol Adherence

A fundamental assumption of this community-based trial is that changes in cessation rates are related to COMMIT-fostered changes in the community environment. It is necessary to examine changes in cessation rates relative both to changes in community environments in the intervention versus comparison communities, and to success of COMMIT activities in intervention communities. The Project Archives supplement the survey-based measures of outcomes and individual-level data on the community environment by focusing on differences and similarities in the implementation of intervention activities. For example, one trial impact objective for health care providers is to have physicians advise their patients to set a "quit date." The surveys of physicians and smokers will provide counts for assessing success in meeting that objective, whereas Program Records will document the activities used to train physicians to give such advice, including the number of trainings that were offered, how many physicians attended, and how long the trainings took. Forms and minutes in the Quarterly Reports may give information about qualitative aspects of specific trainings, e.g., reports of a well received motivational talk, charismatic speaker, or lackluster session. From an examination of all these data relative to both trial-wide and site-specific outcomes, conclusions can be drawn about the aspects of activities that might enhance physician actions in advising smokers to set a quit date.

Reductions in smoking rates and cessation by subgroups of smokers (heavy smokers versus light to moderate smokers) may differ by site. Evaluation will examine outcome differences among sites, including baseline differences in sites (e.g., local media outlets), differences in the population of smokers across sites (e.g., ethnic distribution), and the possibility that specific interventions have had differential success across communities (e.g., variation in the number and types of people recruited for participation in training and policy seminars, the extent of media campaigns, the scope and reach of magnet events, the types of "quit opportunities" provided, the content of newsletters). Assessments will be made of the relationship of cessation outcomes to various summary scores generated by the Program Records System (e.g., overall scores, scores specific to task force activity, etc.), and to other variables constructed from the qualitative data contained in the Quarterly Reports. For example, it will be possible to examine the timeline for completion of mandated activities over the four-year intervention period in relationship to outcomes defined from the survey data. Since the model for change in COMMIT assumes a cooperative effect of multiple activities on outcomes, summary constructs reflecting completion of protocol-mandated activities are appropriate bases for analyses.

The Relationship of Outcome Differences across Sites to Mobilization and Other Process Factors

Sites are likely to vary in the degree of success they have with intervention because of qualitative aspects of the program's delivery, content, and context. Some of these process factors are internal to the project in the communities (e.g., the community mobilization process), while others pertain to external elements in the community context, which exist or occur regardless of the presence of COMMIT.

The community analyses at baseline revealed variation which is important for understanding internal and external factors influencing the mobilization process.

Some communities, for example, had a long history of coalition-building and grassroots activities, while others had little experience in working together as a community on a social issue. This "experience factor" may have an influence on the length of time required for communities to mobilize around the smoking issue and may thus affect the trial outcome [5]. Similarly, there appeared to be great diversity among the communities in the structures available to support and encourage smoking cessation. Some communities, for instance, had few smoking cessation providers and low visibility of the major health voluntary organizations that promote smoking cessation, while others had many more smoking cessation resources and service providers. Communities with few prior structures for provision of cessation services may have difficulty meeting the trial's early targets, if not the long-term smoking cessation goals. Noting and recoding such differences will make it possible to link trial outcome results with such unique "baseline" characteristics of the diverse communities.

Variation in mobilization across sites over the course of intervention will be identified through the information and local interpretations in the Quarterly Reports and other pieces of the Project Archives. Aspects of local organizational structures, site-specific management plans, board composition, interactional dynamics of staff and volunteers, arrangements with the eleven overseeing research institutions, and other internal process factors which have been coded for monitoring purposes will also be examined for their relationships to outcomes.

Community factors external to COMMIT, such as the existence of competing community issues and agendas, also affect the potential for achieving process objectives and project outcomes. For example, the profusion of community health promotion projects in the Vallejo, California, intervention site contributes to difficulties in getting free media attention, since all the projects vie for coverage by the same resource, the sole local newspaper. Social, political, and economic structures may also influence the course of and decisions within the project. The configuration of organizations and worksites varies across the communities; a site characterized by a great many large businesses requires a different strategy for delivery of interventions than a site with workplaces that are mostly small.

Tobacco control messages and activities may meet with different reception in different locales. Information is available in the Quarterly Reports forms on the community context, competing issues, and levels of resistance by local organizations. The Raleigh, North Carolina, site, located in "tobacco country," has experienced the influence of the tobacco industry on participants in COMMIT. Some representatives of local businesses, civic groups, and churches declined to participate, saying things such as "Our Board of Directors includes tobacco farmers" or "This church was build on tobacco money." In a number of sites, some members of task forces and boards have said they wish to avoid confrontation and controversy, to maintain good personal and business relationships in their communities. Such a concern has implications for how activities are carried out and what messages are put into the community through project materials and the media, and ultimately for the outcomes of activities.

The challenge for monitoring and evaluation is to discern not only what else is going on, but which of those events and trends are important. The data are regularly reviewed to identify important variables; assessment of their relationship to trial outcomes awaits the endpoint data. Monitoring of process will facilitate the assessment of variability among sites both for analytic purposes and the development of "how to" information for other, future community projects. Process evaluation is potentially relevant not merely to account for differences among sites at the end of the trial, but to the development of an efficient, generalizable model and the preparation of recommendations for future community studies.

CONCLUSION

COMMIT is introducing interventions into complex social systems, communities, with the intent of motivating local leaders and organizations to direct activities that change the sociocultural environment to produce reductions in smoking behavior. Adherence to a standardized protocol across sites is necessary to preserve experimental integrity, but there is some localization of interventions and thus, protocol implementation and effects may vary. Variation is anticipated as the result of deliberate customizing of activities to fit local conditions, the result of external trends and influences, the dynamics of interpersonal relations among paid and volunteer staff, and a plethora of other unanticipated happenings that occur routinely in communities. These local factors are not necessarily "noise" through which the experimental effect will be detectable by conventional methods; they are essential elements of the trial. The interpretation and generalization of results depends on reliable, valid monitoring of these influences and processes. The system developed in COMMIT for this kind of comprehensive evaluation is both a prototype and a testing ground for a new generation of methods.

REFERENCES

1. G. Sorensen, R. E. Glasgow, and K. Corbett, Promoting Smoking Control through Worksites in the Community Intervention Trial for Smoking Cessation (COMMIT), *International Quarterly of Community Health Education, 11*:3, pp. 239-257, 1990-91.
2. J. K. Ockene, E. L. Lindsay, L. Berger, and N. Hymowitz, Health Care Providers as Key Change Agents in the Community Intervention Trial for Smoking Cessation (COMMIT), *International Quarterly of Community Health Education, 11*:3, pp. 223-237, 1990-91.
3. P. Pomrehn, R. Sciandra, R. Shipley, W. Lynn, and H. Lando, Enhancing Resources for Smoking Cessation through Community Intervention: COMMIT as Prototype, *International Quarterly of Community Health Education, 11*:3, pp. 259-269, 1990-91.

4. L. Wallack and R. Sciandra, Media Advocacy and Public Education in the Community Intervention Trial for Smoking Cessation (COMMIT), *International Quarterly of Community Health Education, 11*:3, pp. 205-222, 1990-91.
5. B. Thompson, L. Wallack, E. Lichtenstein, and T. Pechacek, Principles of Community Organization and Partnership for Smoking Cessation in the Community Intervention Trial for Smoking Cessation (COMMIT), *International Quarterly of Community Health Education, 11*:3, pp. 187-203, 1990-91.
6. J. A. King, L. L. Morris, and C. T. Fitz-Gibbon, *How to Assess Program Implementation*, Sage, Newbury Park, California, 1987.
7. P. H. Rossi and H. E. Freeman, *Evaluation: A Systematic Approach*, (4th Edition), Sage, Newbury Park, California, 1989.
8. J. E. Veney and A. D. Kaluzny, *Evaluation and Decision Making for Health Services Programs*, Prentice Hall, Englewood Cliffs, New Jersey, 1984.
9. E. A. Suchman, *Evaluative Research: Principles and Practice in Public Service and Social Action Programs*, Russell Sage Foundation, New York, 1967.
10. M. Q. Patton, *Qualitative Evaluation and Research Methods*, (2nd Edition), Sage, Newbury Park, California, 1990.
11. M. E. Mattson, K. M. Cummings, W. R. Lynn, C. Giffen, D. Corle, and T. Pechacek, Evaluation Plan for the Community Intervention Trial for Smoking Cessation (COMMIT), *International Quarterly of Community Health Education, 11*:3, pp. 271-290, 1990-91.
12. N. Bracht, K. Corbett, and B. Thompson, *The COMMIT Community Mobilization Experience: Report of a Trial-Wide Study*, Report prepared for the National Cancer Institute and the COMMIT Steering Committee, 1990.
13. K. Lewin, *Field Theory in Social Science*, Harper, New York, 1951.
14. L. Wallack and N. Wallerstein, Health Education and Prevention: Designing Community Initiatives, *International Quarterly of Community Health Education, 7*:4, pp. 319-342, 1986-87.
15. J. Brewer and A. Hunter, *Multimethod Research: A Synthesis of Styles*, Sage, Newbury Park, California, 1989.
16. M. B. Miles and A. M. Huberman, *Qualitative Data Analysis: A Sourcebook of New Methods*, Sage, Newbury Park, California, 1984.

Direct reprint requests to:

Dr. Kitty Corbett
Division of Research
Kaiser Permanente Medical Care Program
3451 Piedmont Avenue
Oakland, CA 94611

BAYWOOD JOURNALS — 1991

ABSTRACTS IN ANTHROPOLOGY**
Covers the four subfields of anthropology: archaeology, linguistics, cultural, and physical anthropology. Indexed cumulatively per volume within the two volume group. Institutional Rate $239.00

A CURRENT BIBLIOGRAPHY ON AFRICAN AFFAIRS*
Provides coverage of published and forthcoming literature on Africana and related subjects. Book reviews, original articles. Institutional Rate $96.00

EMPIRICAL STUDIES OF THE ARTS***
Serving the fields of anthropology, applied aesthetics, psychology, semiotics, and discourse analysis, sociology, and computational stylistics. Institutional Rate $64.00, Individual Rate $25.00

IMAGINATION, COGNITION AND PERSONALITY*
Examines the diverse uses of imagery, fantasy, and consciousness in psychotherapy, behavior modification and related areas of study. Institutional Rate $96.00, Individual Rate $36.00

THE INTERNATIONAL JOURNAL OF AGING AND HUMAN DEVELOPMENT**
Explores the psychological and sociological aspects of aging and the aged. Researches the "human" side of gerontology. Institutional Rate $137.00, Individual Rate $54.00

INTERNATIONAL JOURNAL OF HEALTH SERVICES*
Contains articles on health and social policy, political economy, sociology, history, philosophy, ethics, and law. Institutional Rate $103.00, Individual Rate $36.00

INTERNATIONAL JOURNAL OF PSYCHIATRY IN MEDICINE*
The journal of psychosocial medicine in the general hospital. Performs vital synthesis of linking psychiatry with medicine. Institutional Rate $96.00, Individual Rate $36.00

THE INTERNATIONAL QUARTERLY OF COMMUNITY HEALTH EDUCATION*
Committed to publishing applied research, policy and case studies dealing with community health education and its relationship to social change. Institutional Rate $96.00, Individual Rate $36.00

JOURNAL OF APPLIED FIRE SCIENCE*
An open forum designed to communicate state-of-the-art advances related to all aspects of fire dynamics to those who implement solutions in fire protection. Institutional Rate $95.00

JOURNAL OF COLLECTIVE NEGOTIATIONS IN THE PUBLIC SECTOR*
Investigates every dimension of critical bargaining issues in the public sector. Arbitration and contract techniques. Institutional Rate $96.00, Individual Rate $36.00

JOURNAL OF DRUG EDUCATION*
The definitive journal of the physiological, pharmacological, legal and social aspects of drugs. Curriculum and teacher oriented. Institutional Rate $96.00, Individual Rate $36.00

JOURNAL OF EDUCATIONAL COMPUTING RESEARCH*
International, interdisciplinary publication which views educational computing and its application. Book Reviews, Grant Award listings. Institutional Rate $109.00, Individual Rate $75.00

JOURNAL OF EDUCATIONAL TECHNOLOGY SYSTEMS*
Reports on the application of technology to the teaching process—emphasis on the use of computers as an integral component of educational systems and teacher oriented curriculum. Institutional Rate $96.00

JOURNAL OF ENVIRONMENTAL SYSTEMS*
For those concerned with the analysis, design, and management of our environment. Interdisciplinary, incorporating technological and behavioral sciences. Institutional Rate $96.00*

JOURNAL OF RECREATIONAL MATHEMATICS*
Clarifies abstract concepts encountered in formal instruction. Thought-provoking, adventurous problems for problem-solving pleasure. Institutional Rate $70.00, Individual Rate $18.95

JOURNAL OF TECHNICAL WRITING AND COMMUNICATION*
Addressed to technical writers, editors, and communication specialists. For everyone engaged in the exchange of technical and scientific information. Institutional Rate $96.00, Individual Rate $36.00

NORTH AMERICAN ARCHAEOLOGIST*
The only general journal dedicated solely to North America with coverage of archaeological activity in the United States, Canada, and Northern Mexico. Institutional Rate $96.00, Individual Rate $36.00

OMEGA—JOURNAL OF DEATH AND DYING**
Provides a psychological study of dying, death, bereavement, suicide, and other lethal behaviors. Institutional Rate $145.00, Individual Rate $54.00

Journal frequency and postage and handling costs:
  * 4 issues yearly, postage and handling $4.50 U.S. & Canada, $9.35 elsewhere
  ** 8 issues yearly, postage and handling $9.00 U.S. & Canada, 18.00 elsewhere
  *** 2 issues yearly, postage and handling $3.00 U.S. & Canada, $6.75 elsewhere

Please call or write for additional literature or journal sample issue.

Baywood Publishing Company, Inc. 26 Austin Avenue, P.O. Box 337, Amityville, NY 11701
PHONE (516) 691-1270   FAX (516) 691-1770